TRADITIONAL HEALERS AND CHILDHOOD IN ZIMBABWE

Pamela Reynolds

OHIO UNIVERSITY PRESS
ATHENS

Ohio University Press, Athens, Ohio 45701
© 1996 by Pamela Reynolds
Printed in the United States of America
All rights reserved

01 00 99   5 4 3 2

Ohio University Press books are printed on acid-free paper ∞

Library of Congress Cataloging-in-Publication Data

Reynolds, Pamela, 1944–
    Traditional healers and childhood in Zimbabwe / Pamela Reynolds.
        p.   cm.
    Includes bibliographical references and index.
    ISBN 0-8214-1121-7 (cloth : acid-free paper).
    ISBN 0-8214-1122-5 (paper : acid-free paper)
    1. Zezuru (African people)—Medicine.   2. Shona (African people)
—Medicine.   3. Children, Shona.   4. Healers—Zimbabwe.   I. Title.
DT2913o.Z49R49   1995   94-47391
305.23'096891—dc20   CIP

For

Ingrid Le Roux and Lindy Wilson

CONTENTS

FIGURES AND TABLES

ACKNOWLEDGMENTS

I ACKNOWLEDGE with gratitude the companionship, hospitality, collegial generosity, and instruction proffered to me by the traditional healers of Musami, Mabvuku, Pedzanhamo, and Mbare in Zimbabwe.

I thank officials of the District Administrator's Office in Murehwa, the Ward Committee of Musami, the Mabvuku Town Council and the Harare Municipality for permission to work in the areas they administer.

The fieldwork on which this book is based was done while I was a fellow in the Department of Psychology, University of Zimbabwe. The Research Board of the University generously helped to fund the research.

I am grateful to the following people:

Gordon Chavunduka for introducing me to the people of Musami;
Colleen Cousins for illustrations;
Sally Ehlinger for her skilled secretarial assistance;
Ginny Knight for editing with precision and vision;
Murray Last for criticizing the manuscript;
Reeves Tapfumo for research assistance;
Norman Reynolds and our children, **Talitha, Portia, Sabaa,** and **Abigail** for, once more, supporting me through field research and writing.

I thank the following publishers for permission to reproduce certain papers: **E. J. Brill Publishers**, Leiden; **Kluwer Academic Publishers**, Dordrecht; **International African Institute**; and **Manchester University Press**.

GLOSSARY

The words used in chiShona in reference to traditional healers reflect, in part, the positions in the hierarchy that those possessing spirits are accorded. Current usage, however, especially in relation to western-trained medical workers, confuses the application of the words. The spirit hierarchies include the following (definitions are taken from Hannan 1984; page numbers are indicated in parentheses):

mhondoro 1. Lion. 2. Guardian spirit of tribe (355).

gombwe (pl. *mak-*) 1. Guardian spirit (especially of tribe). 2. Medium of tribal spirit (191).

njuzu Water sprite (474). (*Njuzu* are spirits that live in water and take those whom they wish to possess—usually granting them healing powers—beneath the water to train. They are said to be pale-skinned and to have long, fair hair. Their healing powers are said to be greater than those granted by ancestral spirits. *Njuzu* are classified as alien spirits—*mashave*).

mudzimu (pl. *midzi-, vadz-*) 1. Spirit elder of family. 2. Soul of a dead relative (372).

shave (or *shavi*, pl. *ma-*) Spirit (patronal, as opposed to family or tribal) that takes possession of its human host (602). (They are often described as alien spirits. There are many kinds of *mashave*, some of which grant healing powers.)

ngozi 1. Aggrieved spirit. 2. Revenge inflicted by such a spirit.

uroyi (pl. *va-*) Inherited witchcraft (707).

Various terms are used in reference to someone possessed by a spirit(s). They include:

svikiro Medium (generally of tribal spirit) (623).

mushoperi Diviner (407).

n'anga Diviner-healer. Dealer in medicines and charms (448). (Until recently, the word was spelled *nganga* in chiShona orthography.)

chiremba 1. Doctor. 2. Healer (title with which *n'anga* is addressed). 3. Hospital orderly (89). (The word is often used for a herbalist who does not divine.)

The English term *traditional healers* is unsatisfactory (as is the term *indigenous healers*), but it has been officially adopted by the Zimbabwe National Traditional Healers Association (ZINATHA). Only one traditional healer (apart from the men who sold materia medica in the urban markets) among those with whom I worked did not divine and healed only using herbs: he was, however, guided by a *shave*. He described himself as a *chiremba*. A few claimed to be possessed by *mhondoro* or *gombwe* spirits: they both divined and healed, though one used only snuff and water to heal. I use the term *traditional healer* or *healer* or *n'anga* in reference to all of them unless the context demands greater specificity.

The word *ancestor(s)* is used in the text to refer to a spirit(s) claimed by the living to be the spirit(s) of kin, and the word *shade(s)* is used to describe a spirit(s) not thus defined.

Other words that appear in the text:

banya—round house reserved for ritual purposes.

bira—ritual feast (a spirit is brought out and questioned by senior *n'anga* on its genealogy and intention).

chimbwido—young girl who carried supplies and information between guerrillas and villagers during Zimbabwe's War of Liberation.

gona—calabash or horn filled with medicaments, used by, or prescribed by, *n'anga*.

hakata—divining pieces, often made of wood, sometimes of bone or they may be half-seeds.

kurova guva—to carry out the final funeral ritual (some months after burial).

makumbi—a female diviner-healer, or wife of a diviner-healer, or an assistant.

mbira—a small thumb piano, a musical instrument.

mujibha—young boy who acted as did a *chimbwido*.

muroyi (pl. *varoyi*)—antisocial person who inflicts harm on others generally by witchcraft.

nechombo—senior grandson or acolyte, interpreter of a medium.

nyora—tattoo mark or cicatrix in which "medicine" has been added.

zango—charm (often wrapped in cloth and worn on the arm or waist).

ZANLA—Zimbabwe African National Liberation Army, the military wing of the Zimbabwe African National Union (ZANU).

ZIPRA—Zimbabwe People's Revolutionary Army, the military wing of the Zimbabwe African People's Union (ZAPU).

INTRODUCTION

A STORY about the power of children is woven into one of the central myths of the Shona people. The myth is about Pasipamire, medium of the spirit Chaminuka, who was the foremost rainmaker of his time. He lived near Chitungwiza in Mashonaland and was consulted by chiefs from far and near. Lobengula, leader of the Ndebele, sent him gifts of cattle and young girls. Because he was an "owner of the land," hunters sought his permission to "kill the elephants nicely" and gave him presents of ivory and cloth (see Selous 1981 [first ed. 1881], 331-32 and 1983; Posselt 1935, 201-4; and Ranger 1982, 349-69).

Posselt's (1935, 201-4) account of Chaminuka's life and death is resplendent with the ingredients of legend that include snakes, tamed antelope, obedient bulls, magic, and betrayal. Pasipamire (called Chaminuka in the legend) prophesied the arrival of the whites, saying that "some eight years hence, behold the stranger will enter, and he will build himself white houses." The famous hunter F. C. Selous (1981, 331) described him as a "very powerful 'Ulimo' or god."

In 1883 Pasipamire and his retinue journeyed to meet Lobengula. On the way they were attacked and overwhelmed by Lobengula's warriors at the Shangani River. According to the legend,

> Chaminuka alone survived the slaughter. He sat calmly playing his mbira. His death was decreed. But lo! the spear of the enemy failed to harm him. Perplexed, the warriors fired their rifles at him, but the bullets merely fell in a heap before the intended victim. Even fire—so says the account of another—was built all round him, but it did not scorch him, being mysteriously quenched.
>
> Tired of the repeated though futile efforts of his enemies to

kill him, Chaminuka revealed to them the secret that his death could only be caused by a young boy, sexually pure, who could stab him with fatal results. Once dead, the warriors cut up his body, removing parts of the heart and liver for medicinal and other charms (Posselt, 1935, 201).

The event of the medium's death became profoundly significant and a cluster of myths grew up around it (Ranger 1982, 350). Subsequent mediums of the spirit of Chaminuka became resistance heroes of later oral tradition. Chaminuka was hailed as "Priest primordial" by the poet Chris Magadza in the election victory of ZANU/PF in 1980 (quoted in Ranger 1982, 369).

The legend reflects on moral precepts basic to Shona therapeutics. It illustrates that a medium of powerful spirits is protected by supernatural forces; that individuals, nevertheless, must succumb to destiny; that a sign of moral strength is calmness before danger; that moral fibre allows choice over the means of death; that there is a connection between the power of spirits and the purity of children; and that there is ambivalence and fear in the attitude of people toward spirit mediums.

This book examines the precepts in the Zezuru system of healing that describe conceptions of childhood. In doing so, healers' understanding of the place of children in cosmology is explored, and this entails the description of healers' relationships with the supernatural and with their clients, including children. It looks, in particular, at what conceptions of childhood inform healers' treatment of children and at the acquisition of knowledge, especially its transmission across generations.

THE RESEARCH

During 1982 and 1983 I worked with sixty traditional healers in three areas of Mashonaland in Zimbabwe, where the Zezuru people predominate (for a demographic summary of Zimbabwe, see appendix 1). I worked with sixty healers in three different localities because I wanted to avoid identifying ethnographic description with just a few "informants" in one area. I sought, rather, to find out about conceptions of childhood and patterns of learning among many healers living in more than one place. I selected two communities, Musami in the countryside and Mabvuku in the town, in order to situate the study of traditional healers in the context of their daily lives. This was done to counterbalance what I see as a dangerous tendency in some publications, especially those that focus on healers' pharmacopoeia or their use of myths and symbols, to isolate healers' knowledge and activities from the environment in which it is learned and practiced. I sought, too, to understand the traditional healing complex as it presently exists in a rural and an urban area. As a counterpoint to these studies, I did research among the men who sell materia medica in the Pedzanhamo and Mbare market places, men operating on the fringes of the system, quite outside the web of community relations.

Bourdillon describes the population of Zimbabwe:

> The Zezuru peoples of central Shona country comprise a number of independent chiefdoms, united by geographical propinquity, by their common language and culture and also by some of the greatest religious cults that spread their influence beyond the boundaries of particular chiefdoms. The current chiefdoms, however, result from numerous migrations over the past few centuries and the Zezuru peoples do not have a common history. [Bourdillon 1987b, 17]

The Shona are divided into a number of dispersed patrilineal clans and subclans. The former are distinguished by clan names (*mutupo*) and the latter by praise names (*chidao*). Zezuru clans follow the common central African pattern in being dispersed and exogamous (Fry 1976, 12). Villages are constituted around shallow patrilineages, some four or five generations in depth, from oldest living to apical ancestor. To the patrilineal core, a number of other families are attached by ties of kinship and affinity. Titles to headships of villages, shallow lineages, and domestic groups were inherited adelphically (Garbett 1987, 55).

The first of the three areas I selected is in and around Musami, in the south of Murehwa district, nearly eighty kilometers east of the capital city, Harare. The spirit medium Chaminuka is said to have spent part of his childhood in Musami. This area was chosen because every ten years since 1948 basic sociological surveys have been conducted in five villages there (see Bernardi 1950; Garbett 1960; Chavunduka 1970 forthcoming). The surveys offer background data on migration patterns, land holdings, and kinship ties, against which detailed studies in the life histories and practices of traditional healers could be set. In 1982 there were eight traditional healers in the five villages out of a total population of 1,428, or one healer for every 178 persons. I worked with 36 healers in these and neighboring villages. Garbett describes Musami as follows:

> The villages, which consist of long lines of dwellings are sited on a broad belt of high land between the Nyagui and Showanowe rivers. The main physical feature dominating the landscape is a granite outcrop, Mt. Beta, which towers some 1,800 feet above the villages. Musami lies just south-east of the mountain. The villages are part of the ward (*dunhu*) of Muchagoneyi, one of the wards of the chiefdom of Mangwende. The ward was established according to legend, some four or five generations ago when the ancestors of the present ward head (*sandunhu*) came from the north and were granted permission by the chief to occupy land. The lineage of the ward head is affinally related to Chief Mangwende who is referred to as "son-in-law" (*mukwasha*). The lineage of the headman of Musami village is a branch of the ward head's lineage. [1960, 1]

The second area is Mabvuku, a high-density suburb eleven kilometers outside Harare that was set aside in 1952 for blacks working in Harare (then Salisbury). A ZINATHA (Zimbabwe National Traditional Healers' Association) official estimated that 350 traditional healers operated in Mabvuku in 1983. In the same year the population was 34,000, which allows 97 persons to every healer. I cannot guarantee the accuracy of this estimate, and the municipality did not know how many healers were in the suburb. In the same year, Mabvuku had one clinic, five schools, five bottle stores, five beerhalls, and a police camp.

The third area is made up of the market places of Pedzanhamo and Mbare, where traditional healers sell materia medica from stalls. The markets perch on the edge of Harare city center, the industrial area, the main bus terminus, and the high-density suburb of Mbare. In 1983 materia medica was sold at twelve stalls at Pedzanhamo market and twenty-two at Mbare market. A number of stalls were run by two people. The fourteen men with whom I worked either owned or assisted at stalls in Pedzanhamo, and some also owned stalls at the other market place. The rent for each table was Z$1.40 per week. (A Zimbabwe dollar was then worth roughly half a U.S. dollar). Details of the forty-seven healers with whom I worked closely are given in chapter 1.

I conducted my fieldwork just after the long and bloody war that culminated in Zimbabwe's independence (April 1980), ending almost a hundred years of colonial domination. Communities were licking their wounds and reerecting the scaffolding of relations to support the ordinary rounds of daily life. Each site was an arena for the war, Musami especially: both sets of armies passed through frequently, and each had their representatives among the residents. There must have been few people not directly engaged with the activities of war in one way or another.

I had been out of the country of my birth for fourteen years and returned an alien. For the first year of research I was given a room in an old complex of servants' quarters behind a small shop in Musami. In giving me permission to work in the area, the district councillors assigned me this room, saying that they feared for my safety if I lived outside the service center. Perhaps they wanted to keep an eye on me, too. They had cause to be concerned as, during the war, three black researchers from the University of Zimbabwe had fallen foul of villagers who suspected them of having given information on guerrilla movements to the district commissioner. The three were attacked; one escaped and the other two were killed. Threats of murder sometimes reached my ears, but I met no danger.

During the war, missionaries were massacred at St. Paul's Mission at Musami. On Sunday night, 6 February 1977, seven missionaries were rounded up by twelve young men on a road within the mission station and shot. The missionaries were all white: two were priests, one a brother, and four were sisters. One man survived the rain of bullets, and an elderly sister was left untouched where she fell when the missionaries were being gathered together. The superior of the mission, Father Mark Hackett, was on leave in England at the time. Over the same weekend, five black men were killed in nearby villages.[1] In Musami, after the war, there were conflicting opinions as to the identity of the killers. Some suspected that the Rhodesian security forces committed the atrocity so that it would look as if the guerrillas were responsible.

I watched with wonder the process of reconciliation that was taking place within families and communities and across ethnic divides. In early 1982 I attended an all-night *bira* (ritual feast) and was amazed by an incident that occurred. I sat with the men around a large fire built in a cleared space near the house in which the ritual of calling out a spirit troubling a young woman was being held. On one side of me sat a man who had fought as a freedom fighter from a base in Mozambique, on the other side sat a man who had fought as a soldier in the Rhodesian security forces, and beyond him sat a man who had served for seventeen years as a waiter in Salisbury's top hotel. There we sat at 3:00 A.M.—the white woman, the comrade, the soldier, and the waiter. As the waiter passed around the pot of beer, the comrade leaned close to me and whispered, "He has placed his thumb over the rim of the pot. It means witchcraft. Do not drink from that pot." I had to turn my mind from consideration of the apparent success of reconciliation so soon after a war to concentrate on the ancient threat of witchcraft.

Reconciliation was not always so apparent. One night there was shooting from an army base just eleven kilometers from my room. The next day we discovered that former ZIPRA members had clashed with former ZANLA members. Some soldiers had been killed, twenty-eight had escaped, and three were captured the next day near Musami. Ammunition was discovered near a stream, and we found abandoned camouflage clothes near the village. Nighttime walks became more eerie.

---

[1] Accounts of the massacre are given in the *Rhodesia Herald,* 8 February 1977 and 6 May 1977, and a report on the shrine built to honor the missionaries is in the *Sunday Mail,* 6 February 1983.

Working in Mabvuku was easier in some respects; the war had not had such a direct impact and, as the community was less cohesive, people's fears and suspicions were more diffuse. However, *n'anga* believed that people were stealing their medicines and undermining their spheres of influence, so it took longer for me to gain acceptance. Research among the stallholders of Mbare and Pedzanhamo markets presented another set of problems and rewards. Much of their business deals with sexually transmitted diseases, gambling, love potions, and good luck charms—none of which lend themselves easily to public discussion. To be the only woman among a set of hard-drinking men with witty tongues took some steeling of the nerves.

ANTHROPOLOGIST AS TRAVELER

In pondering the question of how cultural analysis constitutes its objects—societies, traditions, communities, identities—in spatial terms and through specific spatial practices of research, James Clifford examines Bronislaw Malinowski's living arrangements in the field and his style of research:

Let's focus for a moment on two photographs near the beginning of Malinowski's *Argonauts of the Western Pacific* (1922), arguably one of a few crucial texts that established the modern disciplinary norm of a certain kind of participant observation. This fieldwork, you'll recall, rejected a certain style of research: living among fellow whites, calling up "informants" to talk culture in an encampment or on a verandah, sallying forth to "do the village." The fieldwork Malinowski dramatized required one to live full time in the village, learn the language, and be a seriously involved participant observer. The photographs at the beginning of *Argonauts,* Plates I and II, feature "the Ethnographer's tent" among Trobriand dwellings. One shows a small beach settlement, setting for the seafaring Kula activities the book chronicles. The other shows the chief's personal hut in Omarakana village, with the researcher's tent pitched nearby. In the text, Malinowski defends this style of dwelling/research as a (relatively) unobtrusive way of sharing the life of those under study. "In fact, as they knew I would thrust my nose into everything, even where a well-mannered native would not dream of intruding, they finished by regarding me as part and parcel of their life, a necessary evil or nuisance, mitigated by donations of tobacco." He also claimed a kind of panopticism. There was no need to search out the important events in Trobriand life, rituals, rifts, cures, spells, deaths, etc. "They took place under my very eyes, at my own doorstep, so to speak" (Malinowski, 1922, p. 8) (And in this regard, it would be interesting to discuss the image/technology of the research *tent:* its mobility, thin flaps, providing an "inside" where notebooks, special foods, a typewriter, could be kept, a base of operations minimally separated from "the action.") (emphasis in original) [1992, 7]

Clifford goes on to ask a series of "postcolonial" questions about who, exactly, is being observed when a tent is pitched in the middle of a village. In colonial times, "the image represented a powerful localizing strategy: centering 'the culture' around a particular locus, 'the village,' and a certain spatial practice of dwelling/research which itself . . . depended on a complementary localization—that of 'the field.'"
Clifford uses the trope of traveler to describe anthropologists: it is tailor made to fit my experience. He suggests that we view "culture *as* travel," (emphasis in original) challenging anthropologists to examine their use of sites, the way they equate "culture" with locality and their tendency to represent communities as having separate, integral cultures. He conjures up a picture of "cultures" as sites traversed—by tourists, by oil pipelines, by Western commodities, by armies, by radio and television signals. My room in Musami did not constitute a particular locus. I was not a coresident but a traveler, and that suited my task, as thirty-six healers lived scattered in hamlets that stretched for some thirty kilometers along the ridge of hills. The colonial administrators had tried to force people to live in lines, with grazing land to one side of their homes and fields to another. Houses were, therefore, more regimented than they would otherwise have been, yet people still lived among clusters of kin separated from other clusters. I did not study villages but healers in households scattered across a swath

of land. I chose not to focus on healers in one village, nor even in one area.

It is remarkable that the healers accepted me just after a long and bloody war between whites and blacks. I can only suppose that they accepted me because we shared a common interest—in the nature of healing and the character of healers' conceptions of childhood. The healers said that I was possessed by spirits who were granting me healing powers, especially for curing gynecological problems. People among the Xhosa, the Zezuru, and the Tonga have all said that. I have taken it as an expression of generosity and trust and as their acknowledgment of my serious interest in healing. The Zezuru healers laughed at my casual acceptance of their diagnosis and reported to me that, as I failed to act on my spirits' instructions on healing as given to me in dreams, my spirits appeared in their dreams, identified themselves, and gave them guidance on healing and instructions about medicines, seeing that I was too foolish to listen. Had I set up shop in the market place and handled gynecological problems, I would, the healers said, have made a lot of money.

I traveled often between Harare and Musami in a microbus. The journeys served as a transition period between home and the field. Many people accepted lifts, and the trips were interesting and full of laughter, but negotiating the roadblocks (set up to control the distribution of arms by disaffected whites or members of political parties in opposition to the ruling ZANU party) was an ordeal as the microbus was unloaded and each traveler's papers and purpose checked.

Despite not living in one village, I used the participant-observer method of anthropological fieldwork. I spent my days and, often, nights with healers and their families. I talked with them, ate with them, worked with them, interviewed them, sat in on their consultations, collected herbs with them, helped them prepare medicines, exchanged dreams with them, attended rituals with them, and so on. All the while, I was observing healers and children and the relations between them. Homes in the countryside or in town afford little privacy. Most goings-on occur with others, especially children, observing or participating. Consultations between healer and patient are often held in the healer's *banya* (a round house reserved for ritual purposes) but one or more children may perform as acolytes, or a child may be the patient or simply be accompanying kin. While I interviewed a healer, for example, I would watch children listen; while I collected herbs in the bush with a healer, I would observe the healer instruct, direct, or respond to children who went with us. What I learned circled between healers and children. The healers recalled their own childhood experiences, reflected on their conceptions of childhood, and related to children in terms of their practices both as instructors and as healers. The children reflected on the business of healing, the roles of healers, the acquisition of knowledge, and their part as acolytes and patients. As well as participating and observing, I conducted structured interviews, compiled life histories, administered herb tests, documented healers' pharmacopoeia, traced networks, attended rituals, and held many group sessions with healers. I learned much more about healers than is presented in this book; here I have selected aspects of their understanding and practice that deal with childhood.

A PARTIAL ETHNOGRAPHY

The book's aim is modest. It is a partial ethnography. It suggests ways of looking at childhood and healing. It does not present a strong theoretical frame, nor a synthesis, nor a crafted construction of ideas. It represents an exploration of ideas that inform and reflect on practical experience in relationships between healers and children. It is not an ethnography of childhood in that it does not set out to describe patterns of child rearing. As an ethnography, in the words of Stephen Tyler,

> it is fragmentary because it cannot be otherwise. Life in the field is itself fragmentary, not at all organized around familiar ethnological categories like kinship, economy and religion, and . . . [local people] seem to lack communicable visions of a shared, integrated whole; nor do particular experiences present themselves, even to the most hardened sociologist, as conveniently labelled synecdotes, microcosms, or allegories of wholes, whether cultural or theoretical.

At best, we make do with a collection of indexical anecdotes or telling particulars with which to portend that larger unity beyond explicit textualization. It is not just that we cannot see the forest for the trees, but that we have come to feel that there are no forests where the trees are too far apart, just as patches make quilts only if the spaces between them are small enough. [1987, 208]

For, as Tyler says, we confirm in our ethnographies our consciousness of the fragmentary nature of the world, for nothing so well defines our world as the absence of a synthesizing allegory. And in particular our understanding of childhood is fragmentary, and our serious efforts to research it have just begun, at least among peoples who do not live in the modern industrialized nations. Which is not to say that constructions of childhood have not been closely woven into a wide variety of philosophies—they have. Little of this is reproduced in texts that shape Western thoughts—an example of continuing imperialism.

For Clifford, too, "ethnographic truths are inherently *partial—committed and incomplete*" (Clifford 1986, 7). Culture is not an object to be described, neither is it a unified corpus of symbols and meanings that can be definitely interpreted. It is contested, temporal, and emergent. Representation and explanation—both by insiders and outsiders—is implicated in this emergence (Clifford 1986, 19). And it is similar for conceptions of childhood. They change, they reflect contact with other ideas about children's place in the cosmology, and they respond to forces of change, including new systems of medical knowledge and political movements (including war). I offer, then, a partial ethnography, hoping that it will lead to more subtle, concrete ways of reading and writing about childhood in southern Africa.

THE CONTEXT OF ZEZURU THERAPEUTICS

Zezuru healing patterns fit into a system of thought about misfortune and its treatment that is widespread in central and southern Africa. Janzen outlines this system as follows:

The causal premises behind health and disease in this "Bantu" cosmology trace all of life to a central source of power, often named God or some spirit immanent in nature. This power is mediated by middle-range spirits and consecrated human priests or visionary prophets who maintain contact with, or derive inspiration from, the source of power and life. Misfortune, including disease, is any condition whether social, personal, physical, or mystical which falls short of the ordered universe of life—in other words, chaos. Balance between the universe's elements is a subordinate theme, as is purity.

A crucial cosmological notion, therefore, is the distinction drawn in many Bantu societies between "naturally-caused" (God-caused) diseases or misfortunes and those attributed to "human cause." The former misfortunes "just happen" or are "in the order of things" as, for example, in the death of a very old person or in an affliction with readily recognized symptoms and signs which respond to treatment as expected. A widespread range of treatments such as plant preparations, massages, and manipulative techniques are appropriate for afflictions of this type, as are nowadays techniques or modern biomedicine practiced by Western-trained doctors and nurses in hospitals and dispensaries.

In contrast to natural misfortunes and diseases are those caused by chaos in the human world or in the relationship of humans to their environment. An individual may bring disease and suffering upon himself by disregarding social etiquette, ignoring good eating habits, or by turning his back on kinsmen, elders, ancestors, and spirits. An aura of ritual pollution frequently accompanies sickness by "human cause" requiring the sufferer and his fellows to seek ritual purification through sacrifices and confessions so as to achieve reintegration with the good graces of society. Most human-caused affliction in Bantu thought is attributed to the evil intentions of others, or situations of contradiction in which persons are at odds or cross-purposes with one another, as, for example, in the struggle to distribute land equitably from a limited estate at a time when the dependent population is increasing or in launching an enterprise for profit in the face of a strong ethic of the redistribution of goods. Such situations are believed to incur the ill will or envy of others and to lead directly to the breakdown of health in a person, to visible physical sickness, or even to the person's death. This belief in mystically channelled ill wishing operates to reinforce the morality of social redistribution and loyalty to family and kin.

Bantu therapeutic systems follow from these assumptions about the nature of the world and the causes of misfortune, articulating techniques—empirical, social, symbolical—and their specialized experts. Not all medicines are highly specialized. Many are household techniques practiced by parents on children, or by anyone on himself. Yet in areas of life where there is crisis, transition, danger, recurrent accident, high responsibility, or a focus on core social values, consecrated medicines appear, complete with origin charters, exact codes for their use, and the dangers of their misuse. These consecrated medicines may be techniques, chemotherapeutic treatments, behavioral procedures, or highly magical and esoteric affairs. The emergence of a consecrated medicine in an area of life probably derives from the perception that the technique so consecrated, or the ingredient, is powerful, effective, and in need of legitimate control. It is said that "a medicine that can kill, can also heal," and therefore must be carefully used and authorized, the same as in other therapeutic traditions. [1982, 13–14]

There are, in the literature on healing in the region, only scattered references to healers' conceptions of childhood. One, however, is noted by Janzen in a reference to an inventory of consecrated medicines given in 1900 in Lower-Congo (Zaire). The reference illustrates that within the broad system of central and southern African therapeutics, there is a history of specialized handling of issues to do with childhood for, it is noted, areas requiring specialized attention include "a child's upbringing," "spirit children and how to deal with them," "twinship and the parenting of twins," and "origin, residence, [and] identity" (ibid., 16).

Janzen (21) suggests that in giving close readings of misfortune

in individuals' lives, therapeutic movements can be used to understand the nature of social instability, the sources of stress and chronic
affliction in society. They can become barometers of the local human
condition (15). They offer the means for airing dilemmas of social
structure (like anger, conflict, and power) by bracketing their expression with commonly upheld codes of conduct. Therapeutic functions can extend beyond the individual and the hosuehold to society at
large. They can contribute to the redefinition of reality and can imag-
ine alternatives and the consequences of such alternatives if taken.

HEALERS IN MASHONALAND

Zezuru healing varies from this standardized picture, and there is a
generous body of fine literature that depicts the local variance and effects of historical vicissitude (see Bernardi 1950; Bourdillon 1982, 1987b;
Chavunduka 1970, 1978, 1982; Fry 1976; Garbett 1960, 1987; Gelfand
1956, 1959, 1964, 1967, 1977, 1979; Ranger 1982, 1985; Schoffeleers 1978,
1987; and Werbner 1977).

Bourdillon (1987b, 149) describes *n'anga* as traditional diviner-healers whose main function is to communicate with the spirit world.
They generally deal with any problem of an individual and his or her
family and occasionally with the problems of a village community, especially if witchcraft is involved. Bourdillon says that

> the Shona believe that their well-being depends on their rela-
> tionship with spirit guardians who control their lives. Any per-
> sistent trouble or anxiety is likely to be interpreted in terms of
> this relationship and in terms of tensions and ill-will within the
> local community. Sickness is the most common such trouble, but
> by no means the only one. Whenever there is unease concerning
> the spirits, a diviner in touch with the spiritual powers is con-
> sulted in order to resolve it. [ibid., 151]

For Bourdillon (159), *n'anga* diagnose affliction in relation to clients'
general circumstances. The social environment and the politics of the
local community strongly influence the explanation of misfortune.
He is skeptical as to their powers, granting them some success, espe-

cially in psychological cases. He points to the ambiguous position that *n'anga* occupy in Shona society, where they are treated with both respect and caution.

In his analysis of the position of spirit mediums, Fry emphasizes the flexibility of Zezuru beliefs and religious organization. He portrays spirit mediums "as essentially charismatic figures whose creative energy in sensing public opinion, forming and moulding it into support and occasionally collective political action, has a continuous effect on the relations of spirit-mediums to one another and to the lay public" (1976, 4).

For Garbett, mediums in large measure reflect and crystallize public opinion. They are reflexive and reactive but also creative. "This is because there are two aspects to mediumship: the one conservative, traditional, public, constrained by mundane structure; the other, radical, charismatic, personal, capable of overriding and transforming mundane structures" (1987, 47–48).

Chavunduka (a social anthropologist and a healer, as well as the chairperson of ZINATHA) says that "in Shona society the traditional healer is regarded not only as a medicine-man but also as a religious consultant, a legal and political adviser, a police detective, a marriage counsellor and a social worker" (1978, 19).

Gelfand (1964, 23) estimated that there was one *n'anga* to every 800 or 1,000 persons among the Shona. On the basis of a survey done at the end of 1975, Gelfand et al. (1985, 4–5) calculated that the total number of *n'anga* working in all the Zimbabwe urban areas was 4,283, a ratio of one to 234 persons. They estimated that there were approximately 3,839 *n'anga* serving in the Communal Lands, a ratio of one to 956 persons. So the total number of traditional healers in Zimbabwe at the end of 1975 is estimated at about 8,122, or one to every 575 people. At the same time there were about 800 registered medical practitioners—suggesting, the authors conclude, that there are ten times as many *n'anga* as there are medical practitioners. One estimate (ZINATHA 1989) claims that there are 35,000 traditional healers (including midwives) in the country, indicating a ratio of one traditional healer for every 257 persons. That compares with one western-trained medical practitioner for every 6,000 persons. Indicators published by the World Bank (International Bank for Reconstruction and Development

1990) show that in 1965 the ratio of physicians to patients was 8,010 people per physician, and that in 1984 it was 6,700 people per physician. In 1965 there were 990 people per nurse, and in 1984 the figure was 1,000 per nurse.

N'anga (diviner-healers) have often been vilified in past publications about the Shona and still are in current popular writing, in which they are cast as exotic, charismatic, extraordinary people. Yet there are so many of them that only some can possibly fit that caricature. Perhaps we should examine the position of *n'anga* within communities in terms of both their ordinariness and their extra-ordinariness. They are less the custodians of fixed traditions than reflectors, consciously and unconsciously representing the prejudices, habits, and patterns of communities' behavior. They contribute to individual and group attempts to balance order and disorder, morality and immorality, personal desires and social demands.

Some commentators argue that *n'anga* are a conservative force in society. That may be so, but I would caution against underestimating their ingenuity as innovators and their wit in rationalizing change within accepted norms. Part of their brief is to reaffirm the roles, both assigned and assumed, that fit together to give meaning to the whole. As meanings are reinterpreted, so *n'anga* alter their analyses and diagnoses of social needs. *N'anga* currently help make life experience coherent. Their offices proffer resolutions for a variety of familial or communal crises that remain acceptable across generations, sexes, and classes. The healers' role cannot be neatly subsumed under categories of health care or religious succor. It is a role that permeates daily life in an occasionally destructive but often constructive fashion. Traditional healers help patients synchronize the pull between what is good or bad, natural or unnatural, healthy or diseased in the sphere of the spirits, in society, and in self. Their own balance is precarious. They must constantly negotiate their relations with the shades (by nourishing their guardian spirits and by keeping evil spirits at bay); with their kin and neighbors (who legitimate their claims to special powers and support them as clients and patients); and with their own dark sides (to warrant spiritual intervention they must keep pure of heart and morally sound). *N'anga* train as social analysts. Their success in this venture partly determines their reputations and, therefore, income. For, as Victor Turner (1967, 360) suggests, a social explanation for illness is posited.

It seemed to me that in the early 1980s healers were participating in a reflexive moral self-critique. They were examining the past and the character of idealized social categories and in so doing gave flexibility to the present. It was a fascinating process: undertaken in a quiet understated way, yet the moral issues explored were of momentous importance in the lives of individuals and of social groups. The issues included guilt, pain, trauma, confession, evil, witchcraft, trust, ambition, culpability, hierarchy, and possession. I sought to describe their expression as they reflected on the social categories used to describe childhood.

DRAWING ON RITUAL TO HEAL

The research was undertaken in the context of a postcolonial and postwar climate with a clear ascendance of evil in the atmosphere. The weight of a century of colonial oppression as filtered through to children is immeasurable. And the burden of war in which children played powerful and dangerous parts, is huge. Zezuru society had the means to call out into the open some of that pain through ritual measures and the attention integral to healing processes. Ritual (whether in the privacy of exchange between a healer and a patient or in public at a *bira*) has its "own special grammar and vocabulary for scrutinizing the assumptions and principles which in nonritual (mundane, secular, everyday, or profane) contexts are apparently axiomatic" (Turner 1992, 24). With healers, I scrutinized the assumptions and principles of conceptions of childhood that are axiomatic in ordinary living. I concentrated on ritual and practice as expressed in daily life.

The Zezuru of Zimbabwe and the Ndembu of Zambia share in the common system of therapeutic thought of central and southern Africa described above. The Zezuru, like the Ndembu, assume that the living truth of human social relationships should be manifested if the health of individuals or groups is to be sustained (ibid., 27). Ritual among the Shona in the early 1980s did not have the richness of Ndembu ritual as described by Turner in the 1950s. Shona Ritual was characterized by a quietude, a lack of flamboyance that may have been a reflection of the recent past. Or perhaps the understatement of Zezuru ritual is characteristic. It would be interesting to return now and look for change in the public face of ritual enactment fourteen years after Independence. Perhaps the quietude is inherent in the social order; it may even help to explain the success of reconciliation in this area after the war.

The book suggests ways in which ritual provided the means for healing in a newly independent and postwar society. Ritual allowed for moral discourse to be aired. Here I include the smallest items of ritual behavior—items like a healer's propitiation of her ancestral spirits before she searches for herbs in the bush—as well as communal ritual. According to Turner, ritual has creative potential and it encourages a nuanced interplay of thought and mood. "Ritual's multiplicity of elements allows for great flexibility and gives it an immense capacity to portray, interpret, and master radical novelty" (1992, 53). This makes it adaptable to change: it can be the nerve center of cultural sensitivity. The form and content of ritual derive from recollections of previous performances in the heads of those publicly declared to be its masters of ceremonies, and from the flair of those immediately engaged in it—those who appropriately relate traditional components to current social circumstances.

> Here, inheritance and innovation are both social; in a sense, everyone is both author and authored, maker and made. The liturgical armature is the product of past social action; the way that it is bent and stretched to fit the purposes of the moment is also socially determined. At all points there is reciprocity, interaction, communication, open or tacit. [Turner 1992, 67]

That ritual is flexible and that it has the capacity to portray, interpret, and master radical novelty depends on there being an engaged and informed audience. I was deeply impressed by the extent to which ordinary people were carefully informed about the procedures of ritual *even as children* so that knowledge of the tenets of healing, for example, are common while the adaptation to current social circumstances may depend on the brilliance of individual innovation. At the local level, healers were bringing out what was problematic by giving it metaphoric form. They helped to form participants in healing episodes into groups of the concerned. Healers were contributing to the creation, manipulation, and innovation of symbolic and social configurations (see van Binsbergen and Schoffeleers 1985, 7). For the Zezuru, as for the Ndembu, ritual analysis rests

> upon the assumption that what is known, consciously articulated, and confessed before a legitimate public authority, individual or collective, has been defused of its inwardly believed power to harm. When the unknown, invisible, nameless agency has been "produced to view," the assumption is not only that it has now become aseptic, deprived of its capacity for ill, but also that the very energies which unconsciously debilitated the patient, when conscious actually empower him to help himself and his kin and friends. [Turner 1992, 26-27]

It is on such recuperative forces that people were able to draw in recovering from the wounds of war. The "legitimate collectivity" must be a knowing collectivity. Ritual works by bringing things out into the open and this can be a healing process because it is keyed into assumptions about the social, moral, and natural orders. "Exposing to view" cures, but it is not an easy spontaneous matter; rather it is a complex process: the terms of confession which evaluate its honesty and depth are laid down in a cultural subsystem (Turner 1992, 27).

Turner did not write about either a postcolonial situation or one in which a community had just emerged from a state of war. Nevertheless, similar means to heal existed among the Zezuru as among the Ndembu. One form can serve a different function. According to Turner:

> To bring matters into the open, either as nonverbal symbolic constructions or as explicit statements, is the way to undo the harm that concealment . . . , whether conscious and malicious or unconscious and thoughtless, is believed to cause to persons, to interpersonal relationships, and to entire social groups. Thus, when one prays to a shade, it is not enough to make a general confession or to admit inadvertent taboo-breaking. One must specify the secret grudge or problem in the relationship between the living and the dead. It is this covered up matter which is be-

lieved to be affecting not only the quality of the social life but also the biological state of living members of the society, and their environmental conditions. [1992, 12]

The revelation of that which is hidden or dark renders people's grudges accessible to remedial ritual action, to the beneficent influences of the powers and virtues elicited from herbs and trees, from slaughtered animals, from mimetic actions of various kinds. The long cherishing of grudges was thought to lead to recourse to witchcraft; confession forestalled that deadly outcome (ibid., 14). And in the early 1980s in Mashonaland people believed that evil was abroad and witchcraft rife.

To understand the conflicts in the social system, Turner says, one has first to grasp it in its regular operation. (It is hard to know when Zezuru society was last in its regular operation; or is that its genius—to have kept a regularity, an order, in the face of grand forces of disruption?)

Our chances of achieving a better understanding of conceptions of childhood in Africa lie, in part, in a close examination of healing and divination systems. We can learn by focusing on the thought processes of healers, on the relationships they establish between their specialized knowledge and the social worlds of their clients, and on the definition of problems that require their assistance. By examining why and at what stage people decide that a situation to do with a child's illness or distress needs a healer's attention, we can begin to understand the fit between everyday patterns of child rearing and the place allotted children in the esoteric scheme of things. The healer's verdict as he or she resituates the problem within the wider realm of social obligations and the response of kin members to the prescription further reveals people's understanding of children's requirements and interests. These requirements and interests are, of course, framed by cognitive systems that articulate commonsense understandings of everyday life. The systems are expressed in incidents of ill health and distress and in the attentions and interpretations they are given by family members in the domestic arena, in consultation with healers and at ritual occasions.

Healers in Mashonaland were engaged in a series of tasks, some of which fell within the codes of conduct that accompany divinatory and healing systems and others of which called upon their individual creativity. They juxtaposed the use of conventional codes and innovation. Changes at local and national levels required fresh reflection on identity and the realignment of social relationships. Healers had to be cognizant of social structures and of the points at which relationships were showing signs of stress and strain. To meet the challenge, they had to be pure and open in order to be imbued with spiritual force. That is, they had to reflect on self. To have access to the truth they had first to operate on themselves to make themselves susceptible to knowing it—a process of purification.

HEALERS' CONCEPTS OF CHILDHOOD

My prime interest is in conceptions of childhood. As ritual specialists, healers and social commentators, *n'anga* deal with many children and the problems that originate in or reflect on the nature of childhood. Because few societies consciously formulate ideas about childhood, the concepts need to be pieced together by recording experience. Healers handle children as patients and helpers and do so in relation to a scaffolding of ideas about childhood and the place of children in the scheme of things. Reflection on childhood informs us about social relations. Marx (1968, 29) analyzed the individual as "the ensemble of social relations" and Heilbroner (1980, 46) recommends that in order to understand the individual "we pierce the facade of the solitary being to its social roots, and then reconstitute the individual as a person embedded in, and expressing the social forces of a particular society." Ideas about childhood tell us about social forces, and the practice of healers illuminates the interplay between the individual, the social, and the spiritual. Here I begin to explore the knowledge of healers in order to understand how they define the child as an individual and how they describe the social relations that shape the individual.

Working with ideas about childhood calls for an unremitting concentration on the particular and a willingness to follow leads in many directions. Many themes emerged in the research. I have chosen not to impose a pattern on them but to explore some of those that claimed the foreground and to mention others as areas for further research. Themes that were brought to my attention in the field reveal concerns to do with the historical moment. The multiplicity of themes in the book reflect reality. Childhood is not separated from the sphere of adults. It refracts on social, political, economic, and moral concerns. Childhood is a construction but not, as Philippe Aries (1962) would have it, an invention of the industrial West.

The topic calls for a creative methodology. Evidence must be caught on the wing. Part of the success that, it seemed to me, healers had in helping to heal children's distress lay in the flexibility, the understatement, the tranquil incorporation of belief and ritual that they brought into focus in their encounters with children. Those encounters often occurred while other matters were being seen to, so that they were not easy to observe and record. Only some of the encounters between healers and children had as their primary focus the needs or wishes of children; these were often phrased in terms of ill health, troubling dreams, episodes of bad or strange behavior, or incidents of prophetic insight. It is not my intention to offer a comprehensive description of healers' treatment of children but rather to show how the interests of children are enfolded into their practices. I have resisted pressures to be neat and all-knowing in presenting my work; I offer it as fragments that suggest ways of seeing childhood in Africa.

The exploration threw into focus a number of themes. The main themes, or generative metaphors, trace the connections between healers and children and the conceptions of childhood that inform their practice as healers, their relationship with children, and their moral discourse. Another of the main themes has to do with healers' knowledge. A central observation is that the nature of knowledge about *materia medica* is common yet the practice of healing is specialized. In working with healers, I was interested in exploring the nature of the tutorial relationship that mediates the learning process. This finely tuned exchange characterizes the transmission of knowledge between *n'anga* and the young. The quality of the relationship—whether phrased in terms of tenderness, care, attention, laughter, challenge, command, or demand—is integral to the exchange.

The process of social analysis in which healers and children (as healers' assistants) become imbued encourages them to reflect on questions of identity, often expressed in states of possession and dreams. The ways in which individual identity is shaped and the links between individuality and spirituality, on the one hand, and between individuality and community, on the other, are considered. And so is the question of the identity of persons as expressed in relationships across generations—especially in the patterns of training and exchange often shared by healers and their grandchildren. Identity is shaped by notions of morality, especially on the boundaries between purity and impurity, and by ideas of culpability and responsibility.

In order to be successful as healers, *n'anga* must be self-reflective and that self-reflection is given form in their concern with rituals of purification. I suggest that the construction of self occurs in part through the performance of ritual and the interpretation of dreams from, sometimes, an early age. I suggest, too, that healers have to cope with shifts in their clients' perceptions of them as local, trusted guides or as strangers—in both they are the objects of both reverence and ambivalence.

I also examined what healers and children learn about flora and fauna. The flora of Zimbabwe contains more than 5,000 species of flowering plants and ferns; of those about 1,000 have vernacular names. The plants that have been positively identified as being used medically number about 500, or 10 percent of the total flora (Gelfand et al. 1985, 76). These facts present one with a conundrum. Within the bewildering array of species, traditional healers use up to 500 yet, they say, they are not taught how to find them, identify them, gather them, prepare them as medicaments (often combining as many as five ingredients), diagnose illness, or prescribe.[2]

There is neither an apprenticeship nor a formal learning structure. How and when is such an extensive body of knowledge acquired? I

---

[2]In a report on the herbal medicine trade in Natal and Kwazulu, Anthony Cunningham (1988, 22–33) records that over 400 indigenous and 20 exotic species are commercially sold; these species represent 109 different families and all plant forms, from canopy trees to parasitic plants. Cunningham testifies to the wide extent and accuracy of traders' knowledge of medicinal plant resources. He believes that the situation is similar in Zimbabwe.

explore the assumption that healers draw on a body of knowledge accumulated in childhood while living and working with healers in the family, although people strenuously deny that an exchange occurs between healers of different generations or among colleagues.

Another theme, one placed in the foreground by the moment in history, touches on war and the consequent trauma for children. Here, the flexibility of ritual and codes of conduct as handled by healers is a central thread. It is remarkable that healers were able to use ritual innovatively to call out young people's pain and attend to their distress. They were able to draw family and community members into groups that expressed concern for the crises of the young, obliging them to become involved. This contrasts with, I suspect, the rejection and isolation that many young people experience after having suffered trauma during war. Research shows that a major factor affecting children's ability to cope with the effects of trauma is the welfare of the adults with whom they live (see Swartz and Levett 1989, 743). Healers dealt with individual *and* community problems after the wars. In drawing distress into the open, in negotiating reconciliation between families, in incorporating children's problems into communal ritual, healers were able to create a restorative climate.

Evil is a theme in this book and one that, like trauma after war, emerged because of the historical moment. People's experiences during a century of colonialism and a decade of war had, perhaps, given concepts of evil an ascendancy. It was not an easy topic to research and I have written about it using *The Turn of the Screw* by Henry James as it helped to coalesce my understanding of Zezuru ideas about evil. Evil is a topic seldom examined in the literature on healing or on childhood (the volume edited by Parkin [1985] is a notable exception). Chapter 4 is a playful interpretation from the cultural perspective of the other.

ANTICIPATING MISREADINGS

Tyler, in a parody of Bloom, says that "the meaning of the text is the sum of its misreadings." The text cannot dictate its interpretation, for it cannot control the power of its readers:

They respond to a text out of various states of ignorance, irreceptivity, disbelief, and hypersensitivity to form. They are immune in the first extreme to any nuance of form, reading through it, not by means of it, unconscious of it except perhaps in confusion or annoyance. . . . Because the text can eliminate neither ambiguity nor the subjectivity of its authors and readers, it is bound to be misread. . . . [1987, 212]

Here I attempt to ward off some misreadings. The link between healers and children is strong and special but it is only one of the kinds of connections that exist between adults and children. Their relationship represents one link between the sphere of spirituality and everyday existence. Children are identified with purity and innocence, but the tie is metaphoric—it neither excludes the possibility of impurity and the loss of innocence nor is it the only metaphoric representation used with reference to children.

I use healers' recall of their own childhood experiences, especially in chapter 2, and I am aware that memory molds experience. Healers, it seems to me, compose their own biographies as they live them (even as children) and in retrospect. Their life stories are linked to those they compose on behalf of their patients. "We are natural biographers and, as we exist in community, we exist by composing others" (Gordon 1984, 65). Just as they make stories of their past, so they refashion moments of stress in the lives of their patients. As Heilbrun points out, "We tell ourselves stories of our past, make fictions or stories of it, and these narrations *become* the past, the only part of our lives that is not submerged" (1989, 50). They may be "counterfeit integrations" (Roland Barthes's term) but the ingredients include knowledge of self, normative expectations about being called to heal, and perceived place within the context of family and community.

N'anga are legitimated by communities; they are, ideally, held accountable to the community that authorizes their practice. They participate in the process that leads up to legitimation. And they reflect current norms. The stories of their lives, therefore, may be counterfeit, but they integrate many strands of perception to do with social and psychological mores.

Healers' careers undulate. As their popularity waxes and wanes they need to reconsider their life stories. Chapters are added that relate to personal fortune or misfortune, spiritual guidance or neglect, professional celebrity or disrepute. It is a mistake to see healers as the stalwart upholders of tradition or the last bulwark of ancient values. They are more like earthworms, turning the soil, enriching that which is already given. Healers are privy to people's secrets. That makes them vulnerable. Their relations with others are sensitive, nuanced, and mutable. They reflect belief that is both current and vital.

Finally, my comments on the ways in which knowledge is passed down the generations may give rise to misreadings. I say that many healers began to learn about herbs when they were children and that children learn by observation, imitation, and practice. That may be obvious; what I also suggest is that close tutorial relationships between healers and children are often formed and that it is the quality of learning that occurs within those relationships that gives the young entrée to the specialized sphere of divination and healing. Knowledge of *materia medica* is common, but that knowledge is only one facet of the qualifications that *n'anga* need to be accepted as healers. For this reason, I did not subject to statistical analysis the results of tests given to children on their knowledge of herbs. The point is made without such recourse; many children learn about herbs and are articulate about facets of their culture that reflect on healing. Only some deepen that knowledge and immerse themselves in the learning processes that eventually lead to specialized practice as diviners and healers.

In summary, the book ranges over issues as diverse as possession and healing, conceptions of childhood, the acquisition and transfer of expert knowledge by healers, children's conceptions of healing and healers, war and its effects on children, and evil and society. It is about the nature of healers' knowledge and how it relates to an understanding of the world of children. It presents material on the training of healers and the techniques they use, and it explores healers' own life histories. It examines how healers are identified and authenticated in communities as well as how healers acquire vast stores of knowledge about plants and their medicinal value, dreams and dream interpretation, divination procedures, spirits and possession, ritual healing practices, and disease terminology. The process of learning this technical information in childhood is traced and illustrated.

Each chapter concentrates on a particular theme, and together they offer a series of distinct ways into the study of the world of children. Ethnographic description locates and describes children's situations using a triangulation from different starting points. Insights are drawn from different angles and contexts using a range of techniques to gain access to the inner worlds of children.

Part of the intention of the book is to stimulate work on children in Africa as patients or clients and as healers in training. There is a dearth of literature in medical anthropology on these issues. Very little has been written on the spiritual interpretation and remediation of children's problems. Information on children and on childhood socialization experiences is set in specific times and places that highlight issues to do with identity and trauma. Conceptions of childhood are juxtaposed with conceptions of evil, illness, death, and treatment. Ideas about illness and therapy are placed in the context of community but communities are not seen in isolation.

CHAPTER ONE

THE TRAINING OF TRADITIONAL HEALERS

TRADITIONAL HEALERS possess privileged knowledge. That knowledge offers them potential power. In setting out to discover how traditional healers learn, I tried to identify when they establish their empirical orders and in relation to what fundamental codes. Clearly, over time, traditional healers in Zimbabwe have ordered an impressive body of knowledge. I sought to discover from whom, at what age, with what leeway for innovation, and in accord with what checks and balances they learned the use of plants, symbolic systems, and social and psychological analysis—that is, how traditional healers learn of their culture's order.

THE HEALERS

Systems of knowledge are always in transformation, although the process may be greatly hastened or radically altered by formal intervention. Before intervening, we ought to know how traditional healers have ordered the distribution, acquisition, and recognition of knowledge. Researchers find it difficult to discover how traditional healers acquire their knowledge because the Zezuru have no formal apprenticeship or well-demarcated initiation ceremony at which competence and knowledge are either confirmed or tested. Nor is there a single body of knowledge that is passed on.

I have gathered data on 60 traditional healers, but in this section I analyze data from the 47 with whom I worked most closely: 24 from around Musami, 9 from Mabvuku, and 14 from the two Harare market places; 28 of them are men and 19 are women (this does not accurately reflect the sex ratio among healers in Zimbabwe). The national sex ratio for healers is not known, but in 1983 a ZINATHA official estimated that 65 percent of traditional healers were women. Of the 884 entries in ZINATHA's 1980 membership register that listed two full names, 447 were women. I worked with more men because all the stallholders at Pedzanhamo market and all except two at Mbare market were men. I did not uncover recurrent themes suggesting that men and women have distinctive styles in divining or healing. Both men and women were extremely generous and cooperative. I attended rituals at, and spent many nights in the homes of healers of both sexes.

Of the 47 healers, 38 speak in Shona dialects; 25 of them speak Zezuru, 7 Ndau, 4 Manyika, and 2 Korekore. Of the other 9, 3 speak Nyanja, 3 Hilengwe, and 1 each Sena, Ndebele, and Msenga. Forty-one of them were born in Zimbabwe: 27 in Mashonaland, 13 in Manicaland, and 1 in Matabeleland. The other 6 came from neighboring countries: 3 from Malawi, 2 from Mozambique, and 1 from Zambia.

Those living and working in Mabvuku and Harare grew up elsewhere. In Musami, sixteen of the healers come from the district of Murehwa. Five of the men are alien to the district and six live in or near their patrilineal homes. Eight of the women live in their husband's patrilineal home. Two of those women and another two live in or near their father's home, that is, the home of their childhood. Three women and their husbands are alien to the area: one came from Mozambique originally, one from Chihota, and one from Mount Darwin.

Forty-nine percent are between the ages of forty and sixty, 19 percent are over sixty and 32 percent are under forty. The average age is forty-four. There are no clear differences in age between men and women.

The forty-seven healers claimed to draw their healing powers from three classes of spirits: early ancestral spirits (called hero spirits by

Fry 1976, and referred to either as *mhondoro* or *gombwe;* they confer power over an area or a tribe, or they grant rainmaking abilities); family spirits inherited from either the paternal or maternal line (*vadzimu*); and alien spirits (*mashave,* including *njuzu*—the river spirits). Among them the healers have seventy-two spirits; of these, five are early ancestors, twenty-seven are *vadzimu* and forty are *mashave* (four of the last are *njuzu*). One healer in Mabvuku claims to be possessed by seven spirits; another by four; eight others in Musami and Mabvuku have three spirits each; the others have two or one each except for eight who have none (one is a foreigner with different ways, and the others sell *materia medica* in the market places). When pressed the latter say that their interest in healing and the efficacy of their treatment suggest that they must be guided by *mashave.*

Possession by one or more spirits is possible: for example, a Mabvuku woman has one *mhondoro,* one *njuzu,* and two *vadzimu* spirits. Thirty-two of the healers are actually possessed during trances. All but five of them use dreams for healing or divining, and twelve use *hakata* (divining pieces) in their work. Of the spirits identified by name or sex, thirty-three are male and nine are female. No man had a female spirit.

All of the healers use plants and animal parts in their medicines except one man from Musami who has a rainmaking spirit and heals by using snuff and water. Methods of divination include actual possession, the throwing of *hakata,* and the use of dreams. Some use all three methods and some only one. A healer in Musami, who came from Malawi as a young man, divines with the help of the Qur'an, a mirror, and a calabash. A woman from the same area falls into trances but also uses a glass jar in divining. And a man, also in Musami, spits on his hands and divines by inspecting the patterns.

An ancestral spirit (*mudzimu*) usually brings with him or her a *shave* of the healing class to instruct the medium. (Of the ten or more classes of *mashave* only one bestows healing talents.) A healer may also be possessed by a *shave* of another class, for instance, a hunting *shave.* The *njuzu* spirits are said to inhabit water and have light-colored skins and long hair. They take the one whom they wish to possess under the water for spells that vary (in this sample) from four days to four years. Four of the healers in my sample are possessed by river spirits. The river spirits are granted a higher status than either the *vadzimu* or *mashave.*

When spirits are called out during *bira* (rituals of bringing out the spirit when senior *n'anga* question the spirits on their genealogy and intention), they should name themselves and, if inherited, should identify their positions in the family line. The family of the one being possessed will attempt to chase a spirit away if the spirit's claims are suspect. Each new spirit that possesses someone must be greeted with the proper ritual and gifts must be bought or the medium will be made to suffer. Spirits must be thanked at intervals and rewarded with gifts to ensure that the mediums' healing talents are nurtured and their own health and well-being secured. In this way, rituals devoted to the exchange between mediums and their spirits recur.

Fifty-five percent of the healers began to treat before the age of forty: indeed, 23 percent began to treat before they were twenty years old. Thirty-four percent began to treat between the ages of forty and sixty, and 11 percent when over sixty. In other words, 68 percent of them have been treating for over ten years. And the majority of them had signs in their childhood interpreted to them as indications of future possession.

All except two of them know of one or more healers in their lineages. One of the two who have none is possessed by a rain spirit and treats only with snuff and water; the other comes from Malawi but grew up in Zimbabwe and does not know her family's history. Eighty percent of the persons identified in their families (dead and alive) as healers are patrilineal and only 24 percent matrilineal. Seven, five of whom were men, named healers in both paternal and maternal lines. In all, 94 persons of their parental (29), grandparental (47), and great-grandparental (18) generations were named as healers. Five said that the art of healing went far back in their patrilineages: sixteen members of their own generation were named as healers. It is commonly said that healing powers are inherited from the grandparental generation and not from parents: among those with whom I worked, this held true for 50 percent, but 31 percent had one or two parents who were or are healers. There is some overlap in these percentages, as both the parents and grandparents of some were healers.

The variation of patterns among healers is enormously wide. In the sample of forty-seven, the following differences exist. There is a wide age range: one healer who is treating is in her late teens and another is in her early eighties. Some are men, some are women. They inherit their spirits from both or either of the paternal or maternal lineages. Almost without exception, they have one or more healers in their families. Most are possessed by a spirit, some by two or three, one by seven, and some are not possessed. Most are informed about herbs in their dreams, some are not. A variety of divining techniques is used, including spirit possession, *hakata,* a glass, a mirror, spittle, and dreams. One heals only and he uses herbs; another divines and heals but uses only snuff and water. Incomes differ: in the countryside some earn perhaps $20 a month; others in town earn up to $500 a month, and one or two earn more. Some began to treat in their old age, others in their childhood. Some have acolytes, some do not. Some train family members to help them collect and prepare medicine, some do not. Some speak in strange tongues when possessed (one uses a locally invented "language"), and others do not. Some travel widely, often across the country, while others never go to a patient: one old man refuses to leave his village. Some strictly obey certain taboos while others have none or beg their spirits to waive the rule as occasion demands. Some see Christianity as compatible with their calling, others see it as antithetical. Some claim to have secret remedies; some foretell the future; some demand payment only once a cure is effected; some house and feed patients; some exchange information with other healers; some buy their herbs; some are members of traditional healers' organizations; some become possessed with ease; some specialize; others do not.

The variation is bewildering. Writers of books on traditional healers, however, seem to have found sound refrains applicable to vast territories. Has the nature of the anthropological enquiry glossed over these differences, or has recent sociopolitical revolution wrought such great changes in traditional spheres? Nevertheless, despite the variation, there is a norm (in the sense of an authoritative standard) that expresses the most frequent state in which *n'anga* are to be found. The norm is found by talking to a broad spectrum of people and is reflected in the literature on traditional healers in Zimbabwe.

The norm holds that a *n'anga* may be identified in childhood as having been selected by a spirit for future possession. As an adult, the one chosen falls ill, and continuing sickness combined with signs of spiritual intervention, expressed in dreams or strange behavior or both, call attention to the possibility of a healing vocation. Senior diviners are consulted and a series of rituals is launched to test the authenticity of the "calling." Once this has been established to the satisfaction of kin and community, the person is recognized as a spirit medium.

The description of the acquisition of knowledge about healing is always telescoped. An example from the literature follows:

> Typically a person is diagnosed as a potential medium after a period of recurrent illness during which certain symptoms are manifested: for example, wild, strange behaviour; strong, negative reactions to cigarette smoke, cards and buses, and to certain foodstuffs. . . . these symptoms develop and increasingly conform to a cultural stereotype as the potential medium and his or her sponsors become more and more convinced that this is a genuine case of possession. A potential medium . . . encouraged by his or her local sponsors will seek out a medium . . . of local spirits to determine if this is a case of possession and to put in train the ritual procedures necessary to bring out the spirit and get it to speak. [Garbett 1987, 56]

THE PROCESS OF ACQUIRING KNOWLEDGE

Using the experiences of the healers with whom I worked, I have added details in their training and give the following description of the stages through which many of them passed in the course of the qualifying process.

Childhood

1. A healer *may* be selected by a spirit in childhood. Signs of calling in early childhood add authenticity to claims of healing ability. (In my sample, one healer designated his heir before he died. The heir was identified as the healer's son's first child of either sex.)

2. Special ties are established between a child and the healer, often between grandparent and grandchild. As is customary, the child may have been sent by her parents to live with the grandparent. Sometimes the child insists on living with a grandparent who is a healer, even against parental wishes. The child may spend much of her time in the healer's company, participating in trips to collect herbs and in treatment sessions. Most children are taught to classify plants into three categories: poisonous plants, edible plants, and plants that must not be tampered with because they belong to the shades.

3. This instruction is enlarged on from the age of nine. The healer instructs the child in the identification and naming of herbs. The child assists the healer in the preparation and administration of medicines. The child is expected to help during treatment sessions, including those in which the healer is possessed. First dreams are often recalled from this age and first hints of future possession are given in their interpretation.

Young adulthood

4. At about the age of thirteen, the child begins to collect herbs and prepare medicines alone. He may begin to gather herbs on his own initiative. While the healer is away, the child often treats patients, according to the healer's instructions. Frequently, symptoms of illness are first connected to signs of a calling and incidents of odd behavior are similarly interpreted. Sometimes the child rebels either against the order of things or specifically against the healing call. Refusal to attend school is quite frequent. Dreams are more openly interpreted as being messages from the shades. A ritual may be held on behalf of the child during which the shades are invoked and begged to leave the child alone until he grows a little older. Some begin to treat minor ailments on their own.

5. The process of "matriculation" begins, characterized by illness and dreams. The illness initiates a process of consultation with healers or diviners. The illness may be presented as physical or mental, although a division between them is seldom categorically made. Typically, the failure to recover leads to a series of consultations, sometimes within the Western medical system. Consultations are organized by

family members and continue until an acceptable diagnosis, followed by the remission of symptoms, is achieved. The patient may stay with a healer for long periods, even for a number of years. Links are made between the symptoms and life crises. For example, a life crisis might be related to adolescent rebellion, infertility in the first years of marriage, or unemployment.

6. The next stage is one of actual possession. It culminates in a ritual (*bira*) that is held for the emerging healer at which qualified persons bring out the spirit and question her. The spirit must name herself and authenticate her position within the kinship system. The spirit makes demands for particular pieces of the paraphernalia of healing (cloth, dancing axes, skins) and identifies herself as one who grants healing powers. She may promise to introduce another spirit (perhaps a healing *shave*) later on.

7. Soon thereafter the healer begins to treat in his own right. He gradually accumulates power and respect and a reputation for success in certain areas of divination and healing. The spirit introduces the healer to the treatment of progressively more difficult illnesses or problems. Patients are often referred to senior healers until the spirit reveals the means to treat a wider spectrum of problems. The senior healer often does not charge the patients thus referred and informs the junior healer of the diagnosis and treatment. And so the process of learning continues.

Middle age

8. The healer reaches the peak of her career at middle age. The repertoire of illnesses she has cured is wide and she claims a reputation for the cure of particular ailments. The healer is often a leading figure in ritual occasions, especially in bringing out the spirits of others. In describing this stage of their life cycle, many healers admit training others but deny having been trained when they had their spirits brought out. During the process of drawing out spirits, the aspirants share their dreams of herbs with the senior healer who collects them and uses them in treatment. Again, there is the opportunity to exchange knowledge.

Old age

9. Finally, the healer becomes old and the ambivalence in his status becomes exaggerated. He is widely respected, yet people suspect that his powers are declining. The spirit is seen to allow him rest periods. Some say the spirit begins to leave the healer, who becomes mad. Convention holds that the healer is not expected to pass on his knowledge except as a shade, once dead. However, substantial evidence indicates that grandchildren are trained to assume the healing role after the healer's death.

Death

10. Death is followed by the eventual possession of a kin member by the healer's spirit, often after a period of intense rivalry within the family.

Kin play an influential part in the emergence of healers. They make decisions on when the aspirant healer should consult medical practitioners; who should be consulted (traditional or Western, local or alien); what treatment to follow (that is, which diagnosis to accept); and what family investment should be made in curing the patient. Conflict often arises between affinal kin and cognate kin over how to handle the process of possession and who has rights to monies later earned by the healer. According to the norm, the healer plays a passive role: she is not credited with the expression of individual choice or the exercise of power. She is directed by either her kin or her spirit. Thus, she is a pawn in the kinship game, for her spirit is usually an ancestor. At various stages, sometimes in childhood, most often alongside illness, dreams play a part in the process of possession. Among the healers with whom I worked, all those who claimed to be possessed by *vadzimu* denied having been trained to identify herbs, classify plants, prepare medicines, diagnose patients, classify illnesses, or administer treatments. Each claimed that the spirit informed them either during states of trance or through dreams.

When I discussed the process of emergence with healers, it seemed that their roles were less passive than the norm leads one to believe. In childhood, some healers used the process as a means to express eccentricity, antisocialism, bad behavior, or unhappiness at school. Through the long process of consultation and diagnosis, communities attempt to ensure against charlatans. The process therefore allows for the expression of youthful rebellion and, at every stage, provides exits. For example, a patient may be diagnosed as having a *ngozi* (evil spirit), a family *mudzimu* (not a healing one), a *shave* of any of the numerous classes, or as being the victim of witchcraft. If the patient accepts the diagnosis, she can drop out of the qualifying process. The individual can direct family and community attention onto herself through illness (especially effective in a wage earner or a woman responsible for both domestic and agricultural duties); or by behaving in a bizarre way; or by making direct accusations against a kin member, saying that he or she is blocking the spirit or spoiling its emergence by means of witchcraft. The patient wields final control through the manifestation of symptoms. The above are some of the "factors of recurrence" (to use Turner's phrase) that are revealed in an analysis of healers' personal histories.

I contend that in childhood and adulthood the norm obscures the real nature of the learning process. Probably in all societies the real nature of learning is partially obscured by the complexity of the learning process and our ignorance of the actual mechanics of learning. Besides, a certain amount of opacity suits the status quo in upholding explanations as to how and why people must adhere to the established rules of training and qualification.

Undoubtedly, Zezuru traditional healers do acquire a significant body of knowledge about their culture's symbolic systems (its myths, patterns of dream interpretations, use of colors) and the classification of flora and fauna. For example, of the 5,000 species of flowering plants and ferns found in Zimbabwe, most healers use about 500 (Gelfand et al., 1985, 76). Gelfand makes an interesting comment on Zezuru patients' perception of healers' skills. He admits that he held the belief

> that the *nganga* was considered by his patients to have an inherent gift with which he could manipulate circumstances to bring about a desired effect and that the basis of his practice was magic.

But when I asked the Mashona how they accounted for the

cures attributed to the *nganga*, I found that they associated them
with the potency of medicines he prescribed and believed that it
was the *nganga's* knowledge of the right medicine and not any
special quality inherent in him that mattered.

The *nganga* himself denies that knowing the right medicines
or divining the causes of illness is a personal talent. He claims
that his ability and skill are due to a special spiritual endowment.
[1964, 26–27]

The acquisition of special knowledge is intrinsic to the long, complex, and flexible process of becoming a healer.

In summary, healers engage in a wide variety of practice. Yet there
is a norm commonly proffered, against which individual claims to
healing powers are measured. While there is no monopoly, no guild
that defines membership, the authenticity of those seeking to become
healers is measured in terms of the norm. However, the norm does
not fully represent the intricacy and complexity of the period of preparation that healers go through before they fully exercise their power
as healers. Few attempt to set up as healers without the preparation.

THE CRITERION OF AUTHENTICITY

The following case illustrates what can happen if a healer tries to
avoid the preparatory stages. By claiming that three of his immediate
family members were simultaneously possessed, a man brought upon
himself accusations of witchcraft. None of the three had gone through
the preparatory period before he made the claim. Family members
compete to claim possession by the shades because power accompanies possession and the power can be used in the interests of particular
family groups. Kin ties in this case are illustrated in figure 1.

A man, identified as Father in figure 1, now dead, had five sons
(Sons 1 to 5); the eldest two were ill (August 1983). The third son
claimed, on behalf of his wife and two children, that they were each
possessed by a family spirit (*mudzimu*). The man's elder brother (FB)
has a family spirit that had recently been confirmed by the healer who
related the case. Her information came from Son 1.

Son 3 prepared a ritual feast (*bira*) to welcome the spirits of his

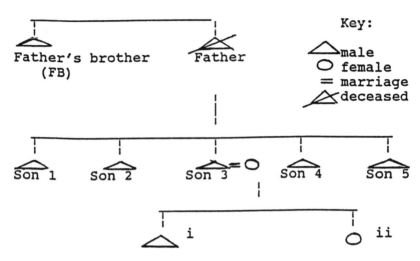

Fig. 1. Kin Ties among Claimants to Possession

wife, his son, and his daughter. At the *bira* his father's elder brother's (FB 1) spirit emerged. When Son 3 claimed that his wife and children were possessed by the spirits of, respectively, his father-in-law (wife's own father), his father, and his mother, his father's brother's spirit challenged him. The latter asked how could he claim possession by the shades of three family members at once (an "unnatural" occurrence), and why was he holding a *bira* for his wife's spirit at his home when it should be held at her natal home? The spirit possessing the father's brother demanded that the spirits speak for themselves. The man's wife's spirit said, "I am the one who breaks legs." The son's spirit said, "I am a fighter. Today no one will leave this house." And the daughter's spirit said nothing. The uncle's spirit responded by saying that he knew that evil powers had been acquired and he warned that every member of the family would eventually be affected and the line might end. Son 3 was accused of obtaining the services of a *chikwambo* (faculty, conferred by *shave*, sent to recover property and punish those who refuse to restore property or to stir trouble, rather as a *ngozi* spirit might) and of enlisting the aid of his wife and children in pursuing his evil intentions. Son 3's wife was accused of causing the paralysis that had afflicted her husband's elder brothers.

After the *bira*, Sons 4 and 5 went to a diviner to request that he return the evil that had been placed on their two eldest brothers to the one who had sent it, that is, to Son 3. The wife of Son 5 asked the healer who related this story to take on the case. She refused, saying that a healer from outside the area must be consulted.

The uncle (FB) held a *bira* to which leading healers in the area were invited (including the storyteller and two others with whom I worked). As he is the senior family member, all kin were obliged to attend. A confrontation occurred when the accusation against Son 3 was made public; the accused son, Son 3, agreed to have the evil in his family chased, thus relinquishing his claims.

In another case a man did not want to admit that his younger sister was possessed by a *mudzimu.* At her *bira,* he ordered his daughter to act as if possessed and he placed her, instead of his sister, on the reed mat. The daughter did as she was told and named an ancestor as her possessing spirit. After the *bira,* she returned home and immediately became mentally confused. Local consensus was that the girl will probably remain mentally confused until a resolution accepted by the whole family is found.

THE ACQUISITION OF TECHNICAL KNOWLEDGE

The term *technical knowledge* refers to healers' stocks of information about materia medica. Many healers know an impressive amount about flora and fauna. They have a wide range of information and show fine discrimination in their observation and classification of leaves, stems, roots, fruits, flowers, and bark. They are able to distinguish plants on the basis of taste, touch, smell, and their appearance across the seasons. Such a range of skill and knowledge is likely to have been acquired over time, under the tutelage of one familiar with the practice of healing. The ability to make fine discriminations is probably not acquired in adulthood; more likely, *some* children are provided the opportunity and encouragement to acquire specialized skills and information.

Evidence in support of this view is given elsewhere in this volume. It includes data from the life histories of healers, detailing their early learning experiences with healers within the family. There is also data on the children and grandchildren of healers currently practicing who have been identified as having been "called," or who act as acolytes, or who assist in the collection and preparation of plants for medicines. To determine whether children who have a healer in their families know more about plants than those who have no healer in their families, I tested twenty-four from each group, matched in terms of age, grade, and sex. To support my supposition that the discrimination and classification of plants begins in childhood, I obtained additional evidence from walks in the veld with healers and their children and grandchildren.

In this book, I shall refer to only one occasion during which children were instructed about materia medica, namely an expedition to collect plants. My assistant and I accompanied an old healer into the veld. With her was her sixteen-year-old granddaughter (her first son's child), her six-year-old granddaughter (her only daughter's child), and a patient's child, also aged six. The patient was a healer too. At the beginning of the walk, the healer knelt by a bush and invoked the shades by sprinkling snuff on the ground. She then addressed them, calling on Nehanda, Chaminuka, Gandera, and many others. She begged the shades to guide her in finding herbs and to grant those herbs healing powers. The children stood before her. We searched for herbs for three hours in an arc from the healer's home. The sixteen-year-old gathered herbs and returned with them to her grandmother. Once, when she admitted to forgetting the name of a bush, her grandmother said, "How can you keep forgetting? I am going to die soon." The girl laughed shyly and repeated the name after her grandmother.

As we searched, we talked and the healer pointed out herbs. She gathered herbs to treat problems that included bewitchment (by a witch or an alien spirit), jealousy, madness, cleansing, the aftereffects of adultery (if someone commits adultery, he or she must, before touching his or her children, take medicine to cancel the effects of the immoral behavior or he or she risks harming the children), anxiety, violence in the mentally disturbed, and physical ailments like diarrhea. She interpreted signs in the environment, like the passing of a whirlwind, as messages from the shades. She took us to a sacred glade and explained what was allowed and what was taboo in the area, and she told stories of the origin of violence between the races. We sat in the glade for an hour, during which the sixteen-year-old searched for rare plants and the six-year-old dug up roots for her grandmother. The woman told the children the name of each plant and its use. For example, when the child brought her a pink, plasticlike flower of an aloe, her grandmother told her that it should be burned and mixed with snake oil (*shato*) and used to treat madness. She told the child to observe that "a mad person moves just as the flowers hang and move on the plant." The child worked with persistence and enjoyment and her grandmother accepted all her offerings.

The old woman told us a great deal. She even discussed with us witchcraft among her fellow villagers. The children listened throughout and watched closely as she gathered herbs. Sometimes she would ask the older girl to find a particular herb or test her knowledge of a particular plant. Our presence rendered the occasion different, but the children demonstrated their knowledge gained from many other walks.

On many occasions, one or two of the children or grandchildren of healers would sit for long periods listening to our discussions. The topics often included witchcraft and its existence among neighbors. No one chased the children away. Yet when I asked healers if they informed children about aspects of their work, particularly the nature of the shades and of evil, they invariably said, "No, such matters are not for the ears of children."

CODES OF CONDUCT AND FEES

Many Zezuru subscribe to the belief that healers are selected by spirits because of the purity of their hearts (*hana*, "heartbeat; conscience"). A particular spirit is said to search for a pocket, a medium, according to two criteria. The spirit "looks for the heart" and seeks a character that will match her own. *Hana* reveals itself in one who is strong willed, well behaved, and stone hearted. Bad dreams are frequently interpreted as trials set by the spirits to test one's willpower, calmness, and strength in the face of adversity. When I asked healers why so many women were possessed by male spirits, they reasoned that men found that women had more reliable hearts and so sought them out as pockets. Thus, in affirming someone's genuine possession during a ritual (*bira*), the community is also recognizing that person's moral purity. In turn, the one recognized is expected to live in accordance with a code of conduct that includes particulars laid down by the possessing spirit, as well as more general restrictions.

According to healers, spirits trouble the children whom they later intend to possess because they need to ensure that the children follow the precepts of the code. For instance, sometimes the spirit wishes to prevent the child from eating certain foods (in the case of one man, his spirit prevented him from eating *sadza,* the staple food, from early childhood), or from being contaminated by Western ideas (as evidenced by fainting in class, dizziness when copying from the blackboard, and other problems at school), or from contact with death (one girl who vomited when anywhere near a funeral was divined to be possessed by a spirit who hated death). Signs such as these are very likely recognized retrospectively; similar patterns can also be identified in the hero myths of other cultures. Nevertheless, I witnessed children receiving such interpretations. Some children whose behavior, eccentricities, health, or intelligence draw attention from adults are seemingly offered the opportunity to claim possession.

The following paragraphs outline the code. The process of becoming a healer involves much more than the acquisition of knowledge about flora and fauna. It involves an acceptance of given principles.

The symbols of office that healers may wear (often copper bangles or black-and-white beaded necklaces) identify them as initiated mediums. They signify that they should not be angered or made to feel anger. Their role is to advise. They should never beat or harm another, even in self-defense. They may not use their power to threaten others. To kill or cause an abortion is considered an act of witchcraft. During the War of Liberation some healers refused to assist either side, saying that their spirits hated bloodshed and that they could not contribute to the war effort in any way. As a result some were beaten or imprisoned (see chap. 3 for details).

In theory, a medium possessed by a hero or guardian spirit (*mhondoro* or *gombwe*) has authority over healers in the area and can punish them (usually in the form of public reprimand or fine). Healers' organizations do discipline members through expulsion or recourse to the law courts. Healers say that the only effective discipline for committing sin is the loss of spiritual attention. The loss dilutes healing powers and the healer's number of patients dwindles. Thus, a person's moral standing and commitment is reflected in his or her success as a healer, which, in turn, can be judged only by the number of patients who call.

While treating a seriously ill patient, healers must keep pure. They must have no sexual intercourse. The herbs that belong to the shades and therefore have healing powers must be touched only by someone who is pure. If herbs are tampered with by someone impure, the one who is possessed falls ill. When a child is selected to help a healer collect herbs, the healer looks for purity in the child's behavior and manners. When someone begins to work with a healer, he or she is cleansed of impurities with water, incense, and smoke. Misbehavior in anyone annoys the shades, even if it is "natural," as in the sexual excesses of young men. Impure persons cannot enter the *banya* (the healer's "clinic") without bringing the shades' anger down upon their families. If an avoidance rule (*muko*) is broken by a healer, even inadvertently, he or she will fall ill or lose the way home. The breach of avoidance rules by anyone may have the same result. A healer told me about an incident in which young boys went hunting. While they were passing through a sacred glade, one boy made a disparaging remark about the scarcity of the game. He disappeared at once and, after wandering aimlessly in the bush, returned home some days later. No one searched for him because they knew he was being punished by the shades.

The duty of a healer is to never forsake others. Some explained their support of the comrades during the war in terms of their duty towards anyone in need. Once a spirit has chosen someone, that individual cannot prevent possession. One who has been granted healing talents is obliged to use them for the good of others. If this is not done, illness will follow, or the healer will receive no more patients. A well-known healer recalls that she was given the power to heal when only seven years old and would tend patients only reluctantly, wanting to play instead. As a result, she became ill at the age of twelve and was taken by the river spirits beneath the water for four days. Upon her return, she healed willingly: the shades had made their point (see the story of her calling in appendix 2).

Healers are perceived to experience advantages and disadvantages in their calling. Healing powers enable mediums to help others. In return, the spirit cares for the mediums and prevents harm from befalling them. However, healers often experience illnesses that lead to possession. And they must obey the code set by the spirits.

Healers are rewarded by the status that accrues to themselves and their families from healing and from access to the world of the shades. Fees are considered as tributes of thanksgiving to the spirits and not as rewards for the healers. A fee must be charged, even to kin, or the medicine will not be effective. The poor are treated free, but if they are wise, they will pay something to ensure recovery. One healer treated his son's child for nothing. Lightning struck the healer's goats and a diviner revealed that the healer's spirit had been angered as he had received no thanks. The practical consequences of this belief are obvious. Some say that the spirit guarantees a cure so that the patient will be able to pay at the time of receiving medicine or later on. The spirit instructs the medium as to whether or not to accept the patient. The spirit does not allow the medium to charge a fee to one who is dying. The patient may be treated, though. Information given by the shades must not be divulged to others.

The code of conduct as outlined above is not articulated as such and aspects of it vary from healer to healer. In essence, however, the code is subscribed to by most healers.

NETWORKS OF KNOWLEDGE, AND THE MARKET IN MEDICINES

In the literature, traditional healers in Zimbabwe are characterized as being secretive about their remedies. The uses to which they put their herbs are considered to vary too widely for a pharmacopoeia to be assembled. Healers deny that they learn from one another or exchange information about herbs. My evidence suggests otherwise. Figure 2 illustrates some of the links among healers that I have traced. Each link represents an exchange of knowledge or of medicine or a sharing of information. The boxes represent the three areas of Musami, Mabvuku, and the market places. Many links exist despite the healers' initial denials that any exist. Many healers refer patients to clinics and hospitals staffed by Western-trained personnel. However, I came upon no instance in which the latter referred a patient to

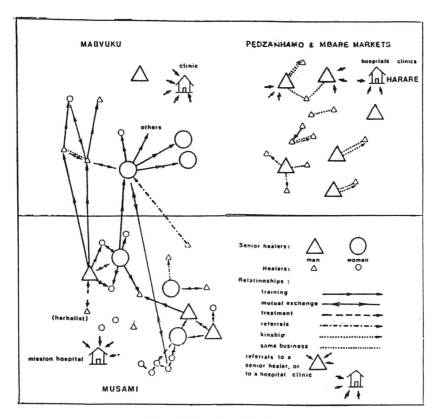

Fig. 2. Networks of Exchange

a traditional healer, perhaps because to do so would be an infringement of the code of the medical profession.

Among the Zezuru, the boundaries between the different categories of healers are blurred. The categories include healers who claim possession by guardian spirits (*mhondoro* or *makombwe*), by ancestral spirits (*vadzimu*), and by alien spirits (*mashave*). A healer may be possessed by only one spirit or by one or more from all three groups. The subtle differences among mediums whose spirits have responsibilities for particular areas or functions—for example, an area or rain spirit—or among healing and family *vadzimu* or among the numerous classes of *mashave,* including the river (*njuzu*) spirits, need not be examined here. They are all part of one system and they share an ideology that is common in essence, but varies in detail.

Organizations representing traditional healers do not differentiate in their membership among the categories. All those who claim to practice under spiritual guidance deny having been trained and all subscribe to the need to surround their practices with secrecy. However, once trust has been established, they are willing to reveal their networks and to share their knowledge. An informant's stage in his life cycle may influence whether he will acknowledge learning from another or teaching someone else. For instance, children talk easily about their learning and their roles as acolytes. Healers busy building their reputations deny that they were taught, but they may admit to teaching others. Old healers often talk openly about their efforts to teach members of a younger generation.

According to Turner (1967), among the Ndembu knowledge is far more literally "power" than it is in the West. Knowledge confers a kind of mystical power on its possessor, giving him or her an affinity with the materia medica used, and enabling the herbalist to activate the latent virtues in the herbs used. The healers with whom I worked seemed to hold the same attitude toward knowledge. The curative strength of a medicine is believed to originate in a combination of the herbs' intrinsic qualities and the healers' spiritual power. Healers who do not claim to be possessed by spirits during states of trance more readily admit to having been taught their knowledge of materia medica. They do not need to establish that their knowledge is directly infused with power from the spirits. Nevertheless, they say that their very interest in herbs and their ability to collect, classify, and use them testifies to their guidance by *mashave* (alien spirits). They describe in detail their early experiences in the company of kin-healers and the graduated nature of their learning, adding that without the guidance of *mashave*, the instruction would soon be forgotten.

The men in the market places who sell the materia medica and paraphernalia used by traditional healers are within the healing tradition, although their role is a new one. In the past, suppliers must have provided healers with exotic objects like cowrie shells, even though procurement from a middleman runs counter to a widely held belief that a healer ought to find and prepare his own medicines. Some say the ingredients must be sought afresh for each new patient (both

Evans-Pritchard [1937] and Turner [1967] give fine portraits of men who exchange materia medica across territories).

The attitude of other healers toward the suppliers is marked by ambivalence: on the one hand, healers in the city need a source for materia medica (particularly for items like lion's fat and baboon's fontanelle); on the other hand, the healers view with suspicion both the salesmen and their products because they infringe some of the tenets of their belief.

The fourteen men with whom I worked in the marketplaces developed their interests and skills in healing in ways similar to those healers in Musami and Mabvuku. For instance, each of the men in the marketplaces identifies incidents in his childhood that were interpreted as hints of his future involvement with healing; each of them lived for part of his childhood with a healer; and each of them recalls dreams relating to his work. I have recorded the stock of four healers at the marketplaces of Pedzanhamo and Mbare and compared them with the remedial substances used by two men living in the countryside. A large portion of the stock of ingredients and their uses is the same for each man.

The men in the markets have established networks that reach across the country and into neighboring states, via traders and practitioners. The marketplaces are also sources of information about variations in patterns of healing, different uses of materia medica, changes in fee structures, and reactions to government measures concerning healing, especially actions toward witchfinders and charlatans. Stallholders proudly claim knowledge of a far greater number of medicines than most healers have. Within and between the two markets, stall owners are linked by kin and friendships. There were no links between the healers in the countryside and the suburb (Musami and Mabvuku, respectively) and those in the marketplaces. Nevertheless, many traditional healers bought materia medica from the stalls, some on a regular basis and in bulk.

CONCLUSION

In Zimbabwe today the world of the healer is undergoing transformation. We have insufficient data to know exactly what healing was before it was transformed. The process is not without direction or social control, although the boundaries between types of healers are blurred, as perhaps they have always been. The difference in the networks outlined above suggests that transformation is occurring within the system in response to particular conditions that affect only certain practitioners, for example, the sellers of materia medica in the marketplaces are meeting new needs and in doing so are adapting traditional mores. The following queries will shed light on the process of change. Will the "wholesalers" in the marketplaces find it in their interests to "qualify" as diviner-healers? Will common membership in an organization such as ZINATHA encourage diviner-healers to patronize the market stalls more openly and to cease being so disparaging of the stallholders' authenticity as healers? Will the distinctions among the roles and tasks of those possessed or guided by different categories of spirits become entrenched, or will they be submerged? Can or should an organization aiming to "professionalize" traditional healers encourage existing variations? Or is a professional organization more likely to formulate a particular philosophy and set of practices?

Most of the healers with whom I worked said that many new spirits began to possess hosts during the War of Liberation, particularly between 1968 and 1972, in order to protect "their children." In the data I gathered from forty-seven healers, only in Musami is there support for this claim: one-quarter of the healers began to treat during a five-year period (1968 to 1972). The number who were called during the war years (1968 to 1979), the ages at which they were called, and the age composition of the sample reveal no particular bulge. Before we can endorse general statements on the increase in the numbers of healers, we need to document more carefully the numbers of healers, their life histories, and the nature and size of their practices.

All but a few of the healers with whom I worked related incidents in their childhood that were interpreted to them as signs of future involvement in healing. All but a few had a close relationship as a child with a healer in the family. These two points suggest that even if the numbers of healers increased during the war, few who had not been prepared for the position joined their ranks. At any one time in a given population there are probably many more potential healers than "graduates." I base this suggestion on my observation of the kin of healers during treatment sessions and on ritual occasions, when one or more demonstrated that he or she was well versed in the lore and rules of the art. Kin often act as midwives or specialize in curing a single ailment; given special circumstances, they too could be called. I suggest that the particular tension during Zimbabwe's struggle for liberation may have encouraged more people than usual to qualify as diviners or healers and that they were drawn from potential candidates well within the complex of the healing ethos.

While the learning process through which traditional healers in Mashonaland pass is neither formalized nor clearly demarcated, it is long, complex, and flexible and cannot be replicated in the curricula of simple herbal courses. Nevertheless, traditional healers are not averse to courses, a pharmacopoeia, or exchange among colleagues. They simply emphasize that knowledge thus acquired is but one step in the process, saying it is not "deep" knowledge. Knowledge not infused with spiritual power is less effective. Ideally the necessary ingredients for accurate divination and successful healing include spiritual guidance, moral purity, a commitment to the client, and the possession of specialized knowledge. Traditional healers cannot envisage a system for themselves in which the acquisition of knowledge is accorded prominence over other aspects of their preparation and recognition as healers.

Among those who are interested in promoting traditional healers as medical practitioners, there is a tendency to ignore other aspects of the healers' work. Efforts are concentrated on documenting their knowledge of flora and fauna and on isolating the effects of their remedies, often suggesting that the healers' other concerns are the stuff of religion or superstition and their continuance need not be nurtured. I believe the various aspects of healers' roles are closely intertwined. If their work is not to be trivialized and their position undermined, a clear study of their techniques of social analysis and the tenets of their psychology must be made.

CHAPTER TWO

DREAMS AND THE CONSTITUTION OF SELF

DREAMS AS "TECHNIQUES OF THE SELF"

IN THE process of studying how knowledge is transmitted across generations I learned something about the role of dreams in what Michel Foucault (1984) has called the "techniques of self" (the ways that people develop knowledge about themselves). The relationships between healers and children (often grandparents and grandchildren) seemed to offer more than the help and companionship that is often observed between the old and young among the Zezuru. The quality of the relationship allowed for an unusual degree of individual expression and self-examination across generations. The examination was conducted in part through the use of dreams.

Foucault (1984, 369) said that in addition to studying and comparing the different techniques of the production of objects and the direction of people by people through government, one must also question "techniques of the self." These, he believed, can be found in different forms in all cultures. Analysis is difficult because the techniques are often invisible and are frequently linked to the techniques for the direction of others. He said that "the dream has absolute primacy for an anthropological understanding of concrete man" (cited in Eribon 1991, 46). This chapter examines dreams as part of the repertoire available for the constitution of self and for the direction of others.

In exploring concepts of the genealogy of ethics, Foucault focuses on the relationship between the individual and a symbolic system:

> So it is not enough to say that the subject is constituted in a symbolic system. It is not just in the play of symbols that the subject is constituted. It is constituted in real practices—historically analyzable practices. There is a technology of the constitution of the self which cuts across symbolic systems while using them. [1984, 369]

Rorty (1986) reminds us of the quarrel between poetry and philosophy, the tension between an effort to achieve self-creation by the recognition of contingency and an effort to achieve universality by the transcendence of contingency. Nietzsche, he says, first saw self-knowledge as self-creation; Freud showed us how every human can generate a self-description. He tracked "conscience to its origin in the contingencies of our upbringing" (ibid.). I trace Zezuru healers' use of dreams as part of their strategy for coping with the contingencies of their upbringing. Dreams are viewed as a part of the description of self.

DREAMS AND THE SYMBOLIC SYSTEM

The challenge in interpreting dreams is to account for the specificity of each symbol and for their shifting combinations and permutations. Dream symbols are susceptible of many meanings and, as Turner (1992, 18) has demonstrated, a single sensorily perceptible vehicle (the outward form) can carry a whole range of significations. For symbols have an aggregative, even cathective capacity. Firth identifies the central problem facing anthropologists interested in the psychological domain as "the translation from individual to social dimension" (1973, 150). My hypothesis is that Zezuru healers interpret the social dimension in constituting themselves as individuals while in the process of becoming socially recognized mediators.

I consider the Zezuru symbolic system as an axis, first in the links among the supernatural, traditional healers (*n'anga*), and individuals, and then as an axis around which the child constitutes him or herself (see figures 3 and 4).

DREAMS AS CONDUITS

In figure 3 the shades, dreams, *n'anga,* and individuals (or individuals within communities) are placed along the axis. The figure represents the play that is made of the symbolic system, with dreams as one point of mediation. Perhaps we can draw an analogy between the symbolic system and an electrical current that is tapped at different points.

The shades (whether *mhondoro, vadzimu, mashave, varoyi,* or *ngozi*) are said to use the dreams of *n'anga* to achieve many purposes. Before I examine these, two points must be made. One is that the shades infiltrate anyone's dreams, not only the dreams of *n'anga.* Anyone can draw insight from the shades via dreams and even draw the power to cure some ailments and foretell some events. Access of the shades to individuals and of individuals to the shades is not wholly dependent on the mediation of diviners or healers. The second point is that neither the shades nor individuals depend wholly on dreams as a medium for communication: dreams are but one piece of technology—"our TV screens," as one *n'anga* explained it.

An analysis of the dreams told to me by *n'anga* suggests that the shades use dreams to call, test, endow, inform, instruct, guide, warn, permit, reprimand, correct, and shape healers. At the same time the shades use healers' dreams to reach the community to diagnose patients, to foretell the future, to call for the redress of neglect, to caution against immoral behavior, and to make connections between the past and the present. The shades of witches (*varoyi*) or lost souls (*ngozi*) use dreams for nefarious ends, to cause harm, demand retribution, or scare the dreamer into compliance. The shades, using dreams and other means, bestow power, but they also revoke it. They are hard taskmasters and take their pound of flesh (usually in the form of beer). People do not become *n'anga* lightly; a sense of unease, of responsibility, even of slight illness is seen to accompany their calling. The shades endow some people with power, yet they offer no security

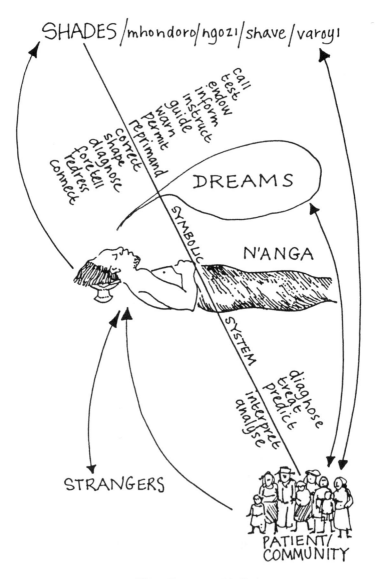

SHADES /mhondoro/ngozi/shave/varoyi

call
test
endow
inform
instruct
guide
warn
permit
reprimand
correct
shape
diagnose
foretell
redress
connect

DREAMS

SYMBOLIC

N'ANGA

SYSTEM

diagnose
treat
predict
interpret
analyse

STRANGERS

PATIENT/
COMMUNITY

Fig. 3. Dreams as Mediators

of tenure. Moral transgressions, neglect, mistakes, disobedience, laziness, greed, or even the process of aging, may result in abandonment by the shades. Abandonment means loss of power and it may lead to madness.

Dreams offer protection to *n'anga* because they foretell major incidents and thus allow the *n'anga* time to prepare for them. During the war, when one *n'anga* was taken by the comrades into the mountains and beaten during interrogation to see if he were a sell-out, he felt aggrieved at his spirits for not having warned him. In fact, while being interrogated he became possessed and, as the ancestors supported the liberation struggle, the comrades accepted his protestations of innocence (see the description of the incident in chapter 3).

We have seen some of the ways in which the shades may be said to use dreams. The norm holds that the healer is passive in that she is a conduit in the process of communication between the ancestors and their descendants. She is said to be the pocket to the shade(s). The process of identification and authentication of someone as a healer is said to be controlled by her kin and community. In studying the histories of healers' coming-out, and in watching phases of the process, I observed that they were actively engaged in petitioning kin for acknowledgment and support of their claims and, hence, for ritual and material involvement. The aspirant healer canvasses for support from among senior healers, knowing that their recognition of the possessing shade's genealogy and good intentions are vital in authenticating the healer's claims. Dreams are used to bolster the aspirant healer's case; she garners them and presents them like signatures on petitions. In doing so she appropriates symbols. The symbols appear in her dreams. She selects which dreams to offer for interpretation. She decides whether or not to accept the interpretation, seeking other explanations in some cases. She decides whether or not to act in accord with the interpretation. It is up to the individual to continue to present dreams or symptoms or patterns of behavior that draw her kin's attention to her singularity and her needs. She acts out her call. Her behavior must accord with her call across time: she must follow the path through a series of variable, flexible, yet determining stages.

Once recognized as possessed, the healer must persuade the community that she has been endowed with spiritual power. She must live in accord with the moral precepts said to be imposed by the shades. She is obliged to treat and should take care not to seem mercenary in her handling of patients. In order to remind the community of the special relationship she has with the supernatural world, the healer holds numerous rituals to which kin and neighbors are invited.

The healer's moral conduct, service to the community, attendance at ritual functions, and performance of rituals are all seen to be avenues of communication with the shade. The healer takes care to make public gestures of respect toward the shade—gestures like taking snuff or removing her shoes before entering her *banya* (spirit's house). The shades are addressed before patients are treated, major decisions are taken, or herbs are collected.

In summary, the shades inform the healer through dreams (though not only through dreams) and, in return, the healer gives thanks and pays respect to the shades, receives fees on behalf of the shades, and lives in accord with the shades' precepts. Using power and information derived from the shades, a healer diagnoses, treats, predicts, interprets, and analyzes. In return for her public services the healer receives respect (though she is often regarded with ambivalence), reward (though she says that fees belong to the shades and she may use them only as directed by the shades), and recognition (though it is conditional). No healer is secure in her command of power from the shades nor in respect from the community. She is constantly involved in a process of negotiation with both spheres and, in part, the currency of negotiations is dreams. Through the dreams of patients and the dreams about patients, a healer has privileged access to others' minds.

DREAMS AND THE CHILD

We have seen how dreams can be used by healers to direct others. Let us now look more closely at the use of dreams to constitute self. Let us shake the kaleidoscope and rearrange the pieces to yield another diagram, the one depicted in figure 4. Here dreams mediate between the child and society and the supernatural.

Drawing from society, the child uses the symbols that clothe dreams

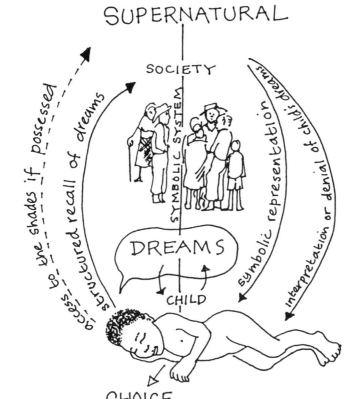

SUPERNATURAL

SOCIETY

SYMBOLIC SYSTEM

access to the shades if possessed

structured recall of dreams

symbolic representation

interpretation or denial of child's dreams

DREAMS

CHILD

CHOICE

repress some/all dreams
recall more dreams
match dreams to behaviour
reject the interpretation
deflect attention
alter behaviour
accept interpretation

Fig. 4. Dreams and the Child

or, at least, into which dreams are molded in order to be communicated. He or she offers up some of his or her dreams for comment. Adults swing between dismissing children's dreams as meaningless and interpreting them as direct messages from the shades. Children's dreams are often regarded as simply to do with growing. Sometimes a child reports his or her dreams and finds that they provoke anxiety in adults and may even result in punishment. For some children this is an early collision with people's ambivalence toward those who have direct dealings with the supernatural.

Sometimes families seek interpretation of children's dreams from *n'anga*. These dreams have already been twice selected: once by the child and once by his or her kin. A child's dream brought to a *n'anga* is likely to be given an interpretation involving the influence of the shades. I have examples of children's dreams that have been interpreted to show that: an ancestor is appealing through the child for a debt to be paid (often the mother's cow); a *ngozi* is calling for compensation to be made to his family for his death that was caused by a *mujibha* (a messenger) during the Liberation War; or a *shave* is impressing upon the family that the child has been selected as a pocket to be possessed later.

Whether or not the family acts on the interpretation depends on the occurrence of the dream in relation to a sequence of other events or signs, including incidents of illness or misfortune. Seldom would much significance be given to a child's dream in isolation. Adults may be skeptical of the power of dreams, especially in children, but many reserve their opinion in case subsequent events prove them wrong. While ancestors are seen to be benevolent and to act on behalf of the interests of the family, they can be punitive and can display unworthy emotions like envy, jealousy, and wrath. In order to persuade the family of their immediate needs, the ancestors often strike through a child, causing illness or even death to the child. A child's dreams may presage such feared interference from the ancestors.

A child knows what interpretation is given to his dreams. To some extent, he chooses what to do with it: he can repress some or all of his dreams; he can recall more dreams; he can match his behavior to the interpretation; or he can reject the interpretation and take care not to participate in the metaphor that links family and the supernatural.

REMEMBRANCES OF CHILDHOOD DREAMS

In recalling incidents and dreams from their childhood that presaged future possession, many *n'anga* emphasize the resistance with which the signs were initially met. The resistance partly reflects the sense of vocation as coming from outside. Parents are often said to ignore signs of possession in their children, hoping that nothing will come of them. They do so partly because possession is seen as a mixed blessing, as has been suggested above. The costs involved can be substantial, and if a spirit is incautiously accepted and it turns out to be a witch or *ngozi* it is difficult to chase away.[1] A family may test a spirit even after it has been authenticated at a *bira* by withholding the cloth and axe due the spirit. A calling may often conflict with a family's Christian beliefs.

One healer recalls that as a young child he dreamt of dancing on hides and of being chased by lions—sometimes he would climb a tree and fall, sometimes run into a river, sometimes fly. These dreams would commonly be interpreted as a spirit testing the will and courage of the dreamer. Each feature has symbolic resonance. For example, the river is the home of the *njuzu*, spirits who confer potent healing powers. When the child used to tell his mother these dreams she would beat him, saying, "Such dreams are not dreamt by children." Later he dreamt of falling stars that would crash and break into pieces. He would pick up the largest piece and jump into a river. An Apostolic priest was consulted and said the dreams predicted the child's death. The boy's mother burned *mbanda* (an aromatic herb used like incense) to chase the dreams. They worsened as the spirit was angered. Later, as a young man, he had hallucinations in which the skyscrapers of Salisbury (now Harare) grew tiny. He could see through cars and make out the parts of their engines, and he could see

---

[1]Compare Favret-Saada (1980, 19 n. 11) who, in writing of "unwitchers" in France, says that "everyone in the Bocage is sufficiently aware of the dangers and servitude attached to magic power to know that it is a poisoned gift which one must not touch unless one's desire to do so is sufficiently strong."

the medicine in people's pockets. These hallucinations occurred shortly before his family finally accepted that he had been called.

Other *n'anga* remember childhood dreams of flying, of grabbing a lion's mouth, of being covered in a black-and-white cloth, of being thrashed with an ox's tail, of being the center of a *bira* dance, of being under water or in caves full of healer's paraphernalia, of black pythons around the neck, and of herbs. Sometimes a family member clearly leads a child in the process of emerging as a healer. Here is one female healer's story: As a young adolescent she began to dream of herbs, and her family accepted that she had been called. Her father was informed in a dream that his daughter's spirit was male and that he, the father, must collect and handle the herbs relevant to her dreams because, if she touched them, she would not bear children. Earlier signs had warned of her future possession: in Grade One at school she would become blind when told to write; at the age of eight she would fall into the river en route to school. It was interpreted by her parents that her spirit was forbidding her to attend school. (This is a theme that quite often emerges in healers' recall of their childhood experiences.) The healer said that she was close to her father. He respected her, as "she had taken his father's name"—that is, she was possessed by the spirit of his father. Before her grandfather's death, he had foretold that he would possess his son's firstborn.[2] And so it had come to pass. After the birth of the son's firstborn a ritual had been held to appease the baby's grandfather's spirit in the hope that he would wait and allow the child to mature before possessing her. When the healer married she bore twins, both of whom died. She said they died because a ritual of appeasement had not been held, partly because she was living far from home.

I have collected many other dreams recalled by *n'anga* from their childhood. Even if the dreams are invested with significance through hindsight, they are informative in revealing the process through which *n'anga* claim to have passed; they confirm the norm offered by society. Or, as Bachelard phrased it, "mediated childhood is more than the sum of our memories" (1971, 126).

---

[2]Berglund (1976, 100) says that Zulu believe the shades can determine whether a child will become a diviner when it is in the womb.

POWER AND MEANING IN CHILDREN'S DREAMS

Some *n'anga* feel that children dream of useless, meaningless things until the age of understanding. This they place at about age seven. However, most *n'anga* hold that the dreams of children are meaningful, that they have power, and that attention ought to be paid to them. Some say that children's dreams are more meaningful than adults' because "their hearts are pure." Jung said that children sometimes have archetypal dreams, which he explains "by the fact that when consciousness begins to dawn, when the child begins to feel that he is, he is still close to the original psychological world from which he has just emerged: a condition of deep consciousness" (1968, 106). Jung believed that a "veil of forgetfulness" is drawn over these experiences, usually at the age of four to six. He continued,

> I have seen cases of ethereal children, so to speak, who had an extraordinary awareness of these psychic facts and were living their life in archetypal dreams and could not adapt. Recently I saw a case of a little girl of ten who had some most amazing mythological dreams. Her father consulted me about these dreams. I could not tell him what I thought because they contained an uncanny prognosis. The little girl died a year later of an infectious disease. She had never been born entirely. [ibid., 107]

I offer Jung's story not to suggest strong parallels between psychoanalysis and Zezuru healing patterns but to suggest that it is not uncommon for children to be seen as emanating from and returning to the world of spirits. As Bachelard says, "childhood, in its archetypal quality, is *communicable*," (1971, 127) and "childhood . . . causes a great abundance of fundamental archetypes" (124).

Some *n'anga* say the interpretation of dreams "is natural," that the meaning is clear, that interpretative ability does not improve over time or with experience. These views accord with Jung's when he says, "the dream is its own interpretation" (1968, 92). Other healers say that making connections between dreams and the incidents that follow teach one how to interpret dreams. Many know medicine that improves the recall of dreams, and some say it helps to make dreams prophetic.[3] The ingredients usually include a vulture's brain and the area around the ear, which are mixed with herbs placed in incisions in the skin that should be pricked with a vulture's claw. The vulture's heart is cooked with herbs and eaten. The medicine is given to trusted children, those with a good heart and an interest in the healing business. There are medicines to chase nightmares and they can also be used as protection against the police.

Dreams are seen to possess an active power. For example, one healer often dreams of flying and warns her husband not to waken her, as if he does she will die while dreaming thus. Berglund claims that "the reality of dreams in Zulu thinking does not limit itself merely to the seen and the heard. It includes the experienced also. Pain in the shoulders after a night of dreams is most definitely spoken of as the shades' activities" (1976, 98). Evans-Pritchard noted that among the Zande bad dreams were commonly interpreted in terms of witchcraft—not as symbols of witchcraft but as actual experiences of it (cited in Firth 1973, 218).

N'anga say that the shades of dead children can enter adults' dreams. Few grant them power or influence, although a senior healer said that the shades of abandoned children, especially those dumped in toilets,[4] can cause more havoc than other aggrieved spirits. They may even kill bachelors, which is a terrible fate as "they [the bachelors] still have their children in their stomachs." In some sense these *ngozi* (the spirits of abandoned children) draw on the power of the shades, who are angered at the waste of their gifts—that is, the birth of children.[5]

Some healers interpret their own children's dreams when they are possessed. Many healers tell children the uses of herbs that the children say are revealed to them in their dreams. For example, a sixteen-year-old girl told her mother's mother (an old and widely respected healer) that, the night before, she had dreamt of a herb, and on wak-

---

[3]Berglund (1976, 114) mentions a plant used by Zulu to make dreams clear.

[4]After Independence, a rash of "baby dumping" sent ripples of horror through the society and has brought draconian sentences on the young mothers.

[5]Zulu believe that children can appear as shades in dreams but they deny that they have power (Berglund, 1976:119).

ing, had collected it from the bush. She asked her grandmother how to use it and was told to crush the leaves into tea or porridge and administer it as protection against witches or sexually transmitted diseases. It could, too, the old woman said, be rubbed into incisions around the navel to relieve stomach pain. The incident illustrates my thesis: that the technical knowledge that is a necessary but not sufficient skill in healing is often learned as a child; that a child can be an active partner in the learning process; and that a child can use dreams as part of the conversation between himself and a healer (most often a grandparent). In claiming to have had the plant revealed to her by the shades in a dream, the girl acted in accord with the norm that says healing is not a learned skill but one endowed by the shades. No contradiction of the norm is seen in the fact that her grandmother told her how to use and prepare the plant as medicine. Her dream legitimized her inquiry. She used the dream to gain knowledge. Unless the girl is prepared to adopt the language (whether consciously or unconsciously) of the symbolic system, she cannot participate in the healing process.

DREAMS AND TECHNICAL KNOWLEDGE

All healers who claim to be possessed or guided by the shades say that their technical knowledge (their knowledge of materia medica) is revealed to them in dreams. They deny that they are taught to identify plants, classify species, prepare medicines, or diagnose illnesses. Every treatment except those for minor ailments, must be revealed in dreams for each patient, even if the illness is one often treated by the healer. Dreams may appear in short spells of sleep during treatment sessions. Spiritual power must be tapped anew for each consultation. *N'anga* constantly tap the power of the shades and the timbre of the relationship between shades and *n'anga* is frequently gauged.

Technical knowledge is acquired over time. The shades introduce healers to progressively more complicated illnesses and gradually extend their range of competence. Recent "graduates" refer difficult cases to their seniors, saying the spirit has not yet revealed the treatment to them. The ingredients are pictured in dreams. In the case of herbs, the whole plant is illustrated and the part to be used picked out. Most medicines are made of a number of ingredients; some *n'anga* say that these are revealed in a series of dreams, sometimes over several nights, and others in the same dream. The dream always shows where the plant may be found but not necessarily the exact spot. Many *n'anga* experiment with new ingredients on themselves before prescribing them. Names are seldom given in dreams: healers ask others to identify those not known to them. A healer who held high office in a national traditional healers' organization claimed that his *mudzimu* had revealed to him an extraordinary set of myths to do with healing that had been drawn from Greek, biblical, and Zezuru mythology. He said that his spirits gave the Latin names of the herbs revealed in his dreams.

As technical knowledge is not taught but revealed, it is no use teaching a child how to identify plants, classify species, prepare "medicines," and so on unless the child is guided at least by a *shave*. Without spiritual guidance the child will simply forget. Therefore, a child with a quick, agile, interested mind that holds information and acquires more will be seen to be spiritually guided. In attaching herself to a healer within the family and in offering her company, doing as bidden, and assisting with the collection of herbs and preparation of medicines, the child is declaring herself to be in communication with the supernatural. The process through which knowledge is acquired is said to be tough—like "climbing an anthill" (*kukwira churu*)—because it requires contact with and testing by the shades. Herbal training courses are thus dismissed as worthless. No healer can guarantee the transmission of her knowledge to future generations as the acquisition of knowledge depends on spiritual endowment. Herbs acquired from another source, even another healer, are often cast away from one's own spirit.

CONCLUSION: DREAMS AND CONNECTIONS

Dreams are invisible to all but the dreamer. Most dreams are discarded. What is remembered and recounted is distinct from what is experienced in dreams—the latter is forever closed to outsiders. Structures emerge in the telling. Crises lend meaning to dreams and the process of self-description shapes their recall. Kuper (1983, 174) hypothesizes that dreams, like myths, are based on systematic transformations. Many Zezuru believe in the reality of invisible (spirits, shades, witches' familiars, etc.) as well as visible beings, and that these can appear in dreams. They believe, too, in the objective power of wishes and thoughts to bless and curse, and in the mystical efficacy of focused social intentions to benefit a patient's total enterprise (Turner 1992, 227).

Zulu believe that without dreams, true and uninterrupted living is not possible. They say, "Dreams are our eyes in the work" (Berglund 1976, 98). Zezuru believe the same: dreamless nights are said to be unhealthy. Dreams mediate between the shades and the living. It seems, too, that it was not only for Freud that dreams represented "the most important road to the subterranean forces which determine the parapraxes in everyday life" (A. Freud 1981, 216).

I offer a dream of a *n'anga* to make a final point: that dreams make connections between personal problems and the burden of an epoch, between the present and the past.

Kazembe is a fairly young healer but his reputation is growing rapidly. He showed signs of future possession as a small child. His mother would take him to the fields and he would become violently ill—he fell unconscious and would have to be carried home. Those were the only signs in his childhood that he remembers. But as a young man working as a domestic servant in Salisbury he used to see antelope asleep in his room. He became ill and a long process of consultation with *n'anga* followed, including an encounter with *njuzu* spirits. Kazembe has three spirits, one of which is from the early ancestors and is the son of a spirit who has possessed ten members of Kazembe's family down the generations. The spirit was instructed by his father to possess a member of the line during the War of Liberation in order to protect the family. The spirit possessed an elder during the wars between the Shona and Ndebele in the nineteenth century.

In dreams Kazembe is shown the miracles that the elder performed against Ndebele warriors. He told me one of these dreams:

> I dreamt of a homestead on top of a mountain. On the steep
> slope of the hill was a stone structure like Zimbabwe. Zulu came
> to attack the village. I saw them beside a river—I saw dust and
> trees shaking. I took a spear and struck it into the ground and

the water in the river turned to blood to prevent their crossing. The whole village began to run away out of the stone structure through small gaps in the walls to the village of Nyamapanga.

Kazembe says that it was a very frightening dream. He thinks the incident actually happened. He struck the spear in the dream, but it was really the elder whom his spirit then possessed. What concerns us here is that the story of the river turning to blood is known in the area and it is not disputed that Kazembe's spirit was involved. Besides, the area delineated in the dream was a troublesome place to go to during the War of Liberation. Soldiers in the Rhodesian army were badly stung by bees; a snake without a head or tail (because it was so long) was often seen there; a red cloth was found there; motorists would travel through at night and in the morning find themselves in the same spot. The dreams fit local myths about the original claim to ownership of the land. The dreams knit together the people's experiences of war. Kazembe told me his dreams just after the War of Liberation had ended, at a time when he was treating children traumatized by their experiences during the war. His treatment depended in part on their dreams.

CHAPTER THREE

CHILDREN OF TRIBULATION: THE NEED AND THE MEANS TO HEAL WAR TRAUMA

> War unleashes suffering,
> It opens the flood gates of hell,
> To swallow the innocent.
>
> —Thomas Mapfumo,
> "Chirizevha Chapera" (see appendix 3)

THE NEED FOR HEALING

THIS CHAPTER is about the unseen world of war—the unrecorded consequences for children of large-scale horror. There are two parts to it. The first is on the need for healing: it is an account of children's suffering during Zimbabwe's War of Liberation and their part in the fight for freedom. The second describes the means for healing: it examines how traditional healers (*n'anga*) provided opportunities through ritual for reconciliation and the soothing of individual trauma.

Although I had not intended studying the aftermath of war, it soon became clear that *n'anga* were at the center of a profoundly important process. Like tailors and seamstresses, *n'anga* were patching and darning the fabric of rural society as it set about restoring and reconstructing relations sorely strained by war. Here I celebrate the role *n'anga* played in reconciliation. As ritual specialists, they laid salve on wounds where the social dislocation was not absolute.

During war many aspects of childhood are denied or foreshortened. After war, children return to childhood: some go with relief, others with reluctance; some cannot return. The second part of this paper explores the process of return.

SWALLOWING THE INNOCENT: CHILDREN'S EXPERIENCES OF WAR

Children's suffering during Zimbabwe's War of Liberation was vast. The pain, loss, and terror inflicted by adults upon children during war must be acknowledged. Adults cause wars. Even when war has a just cause, like shaking off the manacles of colonialism, its true nature must be faced.

In this section I indicate the extent of the suffering experienced by children in Zimbabwe between 1970 and 1980, during the war fought by the people of Zimbabwe against Britain's colonial government. (Although Rhodesian prime minister Ian Smith had made a Unilateral Declaration of Independence from Britain in 1965, that, in my opinion, did not absolve the overlords of their responsibility.)

The data are gleaned from newspaper clippings from the *Rhodesia Herald* (*RH*) and the *Sunday Mail* (*SM*), the two newspapers with the largest circulation.[1] Both were censored and both represented the government's interests. Data are also drawn from evidence put forward by the Catholic Commission for Justice and Peace (CCJP) and other sources available in the National Archives. It was not possible to draw on ZANU-PF records as the party's library is not yet properly housed or catalogued. I have drawn, too, on published writings, especially Moore-King's *White Man, Black War* (1988) and the J. Z. Moyo Social History Project *So That Our Youngsters Will Know* (forthcoming).

---

[1] I thank Margaret Lewis for compiling for me a collection of materials (mostly newspaper cuttings) on children's experiences in Zimbabwe's War of Liberation. The collection will be lodged with the National Archives.

Children's Deaths

During the war, newspapers in Rhodesia relied on official communiques and government-sanctioned tours for their news. Journalists' reports often served as propaganda for the government. Many of the news items detailing the killing of children were released to "prove" that the freedom fighters (whom the Rhodesians called terrorists) were savages.

A quick count in the two newspapers reveals that 130 black children and 23 white children were reported killed. In the three worst years of the war (1977–1979), 110 black children died. They were shot, blown up by landmines, mangled by hand grenades, burned in houses, and drowned in rivers. (Examples of press reports referring to these deaths are given in appendix 4, while in appendix 5 one schoolboy narrates his experience of a brutality many endured.) The number of black children recorded as having been killed is but the tip of an iceberg. The Rhodesian Security Forces released the figures on the number of European and African civilians and Security Forces killed. They also gave the number of "terrorists" killed, which included civilians who were killed for breaking curfew and for "running with" the "terrorists."[2] Given the role that children played as *mujibha* and *chimbwido*,[3] many of these casualties must have been children. Moore-King

---

[2]The high incidence of civilian deaths was deplored in the report "Rhodesia: the propaganda war" (CCJP 1977, 30). Many deaths were not recorded in newspapers or official communiques. The report observes that "civilians bear the brunt of the war. Since December 1972 a total of 1,552 African and 82 European civilians have died, victims of both sides of the conflict. This is five times the number of security forces killed during the war (329) and more than half the guerrillas killed (2,567). Among these deaths are 222 curfew breakers and 227 listed as 'running with or assisting terrorists.'"

[3]*Mujibha* (*mujiba*) were young boys who carried supplies and information between the guerrillas and the villagers; *chimbwido* were young girls who did the same (Hannan's *Standard Shona Dictionary* defines neither word, although the dictionary was revised in 1984 and reprinted in 1987). *Mujibha* and *chimbwido* are singular forms; the plurals are *vanamujibha* and *vanachimbwido*. In published writings in English an *s* is added to indicate plurality. To avoid confusion I shall use the singular form of both words for one or many.

gives horrifying accounts of Security Forces[4] shooting a woman and two children at night (1988, 36–50) and a teenage boy who broke the curfew (63–64).

Trauma and Loss

The trauma that children suffered from injuries they sustained, horrors they witnessed, and chaos in which they participated is immeasurable. Consider just one story told by Moore-King (1988), who fought as a soldier in the Rhodesian Army. His account is given in appendix 6.

As well as losing parents and other kin killed in the war, thousands of children lost their security: their homes were burned, they were forced to flee as refugees, or they were herded into "protected villages." In September 1977 the CCJP estimated that the government had forced 500,000 people to live in protected villages. Cilliers (1985) estimates that 750,000 people had been moved to these camps by the end of the war. Appendix 7 describes conditions in these settlements and the state of refugees, many of whom were children.

Health

Children's health deteriorated dramatically as a direct consequence of the war. In the countryside, farms were dislocated, food production decreased, and services were disrupted. Many rural clinics and hospitals ceased to function (half the clinics in Mashonaland province had closed by May 1979), pre-and postnatal care fell away, immunization systems collapsed, and drugs were scarce. Infant mortality rates increased, according to the *Sunday Mail* (20 May 1979), and disease was said to spread rapidly through the "protected villages." The Rhodesian Medical Association issued a statement in the *Sunday Mail* (28

---

[4]The terms *soldiers* or *Security Forces* are used in this book to refer to members of the Rhodesian Army controlled by the Rhodesian government. The government was led by Ian Smith's Rhodesian Front Party, which unilaterally declared independence (UDI) from the British colonial authority on 11 November 1965. The terms *guerrillas, comrades,* and *freedom fighters* are used to refer to members of ZANLA and ZIPRA.

January 1979) that warned, "If hostilities continue, epidemics and disease will become widespread in cities, towns and rural areas throughout Rhodesia" (for the full statement, see appendix 8).

Education

As early as February 1973, schools in the countryside were being closed (*RH,* 8 February 1973). In the first six months of 1977, 300 primary schools and nine secondary schools were closed, denying 42,000 children an education (*RH,* 30 July 1977, quotes the Minister of Education). By June 1978, 770 primary schools (of which 62 had been burned down) and 84 secondary schools had been forced to close for varying periods. "The total enrolment at the 770 primary schools at the time of closure was 196,682, with 4,184 teachers" (*RH,* 9 June 1978). Enrollment of African pupils was 200,000 pupils below the expected target of 944,000, according to the Secretary for African Education. Twenty-five secondary schools had been closed and one had been burned down. Their enrollments had totaled 6,186 pupils, with 308 teachers. Forty-five black teachers had been killed.

The following facts were given by an officer in the Ministry of Education in October 1978:

> 1,016 schools closed, including 35 secondary schools. 5,726 teachers out of work, including about 460 secondary teachers. 246,000 pupil places lost, including 8,900 secondary places. 78 teachers killed in terrorist activities. [*RH,* 25 October 1978]

By the end of 1978, 25 percent of pupils were without school places (*RH,* 22 November 1978).

Bourdillon and Gundani say that the guerrillas closed schools, especially during the last years of the war (1977-1979) "in order not to put at a disadvantage the many young people who were joining the guerrilla forces and in order to show that the guerrilla forces wielded more power than the forces of the government . . ." (1988, 151).

Abductions/Recruitment

The *Rhodesia Herald* described the first attack (5 July 1973) on a mission school, St. Alberts, during which children were marched off toward the Mozambique border, in these words:

SWOOP ON MISSION

THEN CHILD "RECRUITS" HUSTLED INTO BUSH

MASS KIDNAP BY TERRORISTS

WOMEN, PRIEST STILL MISSING.

A seventeen-man, machine-gun-wielding terrorist band swooped on a lonely Jesuit mission, near Centenary, on Thursday night and after holding priests and teachers at gunpoint and looting a store, pulled out with 273 people, most of them children. [7 July 1973]

Press accounts appeared of at least ten other schools from which children were said to have been abducted. Appendix 9 gives newspaper reports and a teacher's account of an occasion when 400 pupils left Manama Mission with four men and crossed the border into Botswana. Rhodesian sources claimed that the children had been abducted at gunpoint; pupils claimed that they had planned to leave and join the liberation forces. On 9 February 1977 the *Rhodesia Herald* reported that 333 of the students refused to return home.

On 6 June 1978 the joint Minister of Foreign Affairs said that 40,000 to 50,000 children had left Rhodesia to join the liberation forces. The secretary for the Liaison Committee for National Women's Organisations (LCNWO) said that "70,000 children had been abducted" (*RH*, 20 July 1978). The LCNWO was asking the Queen of England to intercede and send the children home to their parents. A nice irony.

Children in Musami Remember the War

Children in Musami, like children in all areas of the country, suffered during the war. I interviewed thirty-five children (aged eight to seventeen) in Musami about their experiences during the war. Of those, twenty-four said that they had seen people killed.[5] They saw people burned to death, people drowned in rivers (their legs tied together), people buried alive, people shot, and people accused of being

---

[5]Four of the thirty-five had spent the years of war living in the city and had neither participated in it nor witnessed its horrors. Only one child who lived in the countryside "saw nothing."

witches killed. One child saw his grandfather beaten. Others saw houses burned down or were forced to watch soldiers of the Rhodesian Security Forces burn the bodies of comrades. Five of the children said that they had been beaten by soldiers. The following statement, by one of the children I interviewed, is typical:

> "Soldiers took boys of my age and beat us in the camps. They wanted us to tell them where they could find comrades. They beat us whether we knew or not. But we never told them."

The children expressed their horror at the killing they had witnessed. They often stressed that the victims were innocent of wrongdoing; no child offered the condition of warfare as an excuse, nor did they judge members of one side of the fight more leniently than the other. They said:

> "I saw people killed for doing no wrong."

> "People were killed for no apparent reason."

> "I saw people killed for nothing. They were just shot like animals."

The children often commented on the fact that those killed were given no chance to rebut charges brought against them:

> "People were killed mercilessly for no reason—merely because so-and-so said he or she was a sell-out or a witch."

> "I saw people killed. For example, one would hear people say *'Mutengesi'* (sell-out) then that person would be killed without even having been proved to have been a sell-out."

Many of the children responded to the terror tactics of the Rhodesian Security Forces by committing themselves to fight for liberation; some were threatened, some beaten, and some bribed to inform against the comrades. Children had to make momentous decisions about how to respond to these forces and what position to take in relation to knowledge they acquired as members of communities caught in the midst of war.

A child who was fourteen at the end of the war recounts a frightening experience:

> One day soldiers came to our village. I was still very young and so was not allowed to go to a camp. The soldiers came. I don't know if someone had informed the comrades—because from nowhere the comrades arrived. They broke up and started moving in twos. The comrades told us to go and hide. All of a sudden gunfire started. When gunfire started we were about two kilometers from home. And then the helicopter arrived. Shots started coming from the helicopter aimed at us. I don't know how we survived. We reached home and hid in the house. Shots were fired at the hut and I thought to myself, "This is the end." But as soon as it had started the firing suddenly stopped.

Children Who Left Home to Fight

Many students left the country to fight with the comrades. Some of these young people were interviewed in 1986 and 1987 as part of a social history project. (The interviews, to be published under the title *So That Our Youngsters Will Know,* will be housed in the Zimbabwe archives.) The following excerpts illustrate the reasons why young people left to join the liberation forces and the hardship they suffered in doing so.

Again and again the major cause of their going is said to have been the brutality of the Rhodesian Security Forces.

> I left home after I had seen the terrible killing of the people by the regime. People were shot dead in public places, in front of their children and wives. A certain man who lived near us was shot dead at a beer gathering. His dead body was then carried uncovered on the back of a pick-up. The dead man's mother and wife were shown the corpse, and it was taken to the police station. It was then put on a table outside the police yard for some days. This touched me so much that I left straightaway to cross the Botswana border. [Partson Ndou of Beitbridge]

> What caused me to go for struggle most of all was that one day I found the next door house being burned and people receiv-

ing brutal kicks, even the baby. They did not ask, Where do you come from? but simply beat you and tortured you. My father was again tortured and beaten. My sister, young brothers, and even my baby sister were beaten. I chose the decision that I had better die than be treated badly in my mother country. We were about three dozens and it was a night journey. . . . really, my aim was to come back soon and fight the Rhodesian Front. [Daniel Mpofu]

Another interviewee reflects on the difficulties of the journey out of the country:

Among us all, none was clever enough to lead us. So we kept asking each other where to go. After wasting some hours we agreed among ourselves that we would look for some place where we could get directions. We carried on further until we found a well-built house, which seemed to be a store. We didn't hesitate but went straight toward the home. As we approached we noticed about fifteen boys and girls grouped around another big house which was painted white. By the time we entered the home we were welcomed by two armed brothers who directed us to the group of boys and girls.

By that time it was midday. We were given food to eat. After eating I felt like sleeping, but I was told we should move quickly because there was still a long way to go. Really, I was weak and didn't want to move, but as I thought of dropping out and going back, I got a mental picture of bullets flying at me.

We departed at 5:00 p.m. and we walked about three or four kilometers, when a helicopter flew over us. Fortunately we were walking with guerrillas who commanded us not to run but to stretch ourselves down. We protected ourselves under rocks, and stayed until we were told to move, as by now the helicopter had passed us. We were also told that the man who had welcomed us was the one who reported our presence. Two of the guerrillas went back in a fury. They brought the man, and killed him, which I did not expect. We walked three nights and three days until we reached the border. [Adwell Ndlovu]

Once in the camps the young people suffered harsh conditions and often longed for home:

There was military life and no holidays, only weekends. I learnt that in a war you must stay vigilant and you must be prepared for anything that may come at any time. When I was in Zambia, in the first days I could only think about my father and mother at home. [Stanley Ndlovu]

We had settled in a place [in Solwezi, Zambia] that had many tsetse flies and mosquitoes. Some of us became seriously ill, but the surprising thing was that all of us were ready to sacrifice in the fight against the regime. Bombardments came in Solwezi in 1979, several times. We lost many comrades when bombardments took place. We had to vanish into the bush for about a week, eating food at night. Then we would spend a week drinking tea, without a piece of bread even. The weaker ones died before the end of the week. I felt so much sympathy when I fixed my eyes on my weaker fellows who failed to get up because of hunger. Some were weakened by disease spread by mosquitoes. [Roger Ndiweni]

At J. Z. [Moyo, a camp in Zambia] there were too many people. Now the situation was very hard because there was no good accommodation. We slept under trees. There was a water shortage, and you could only wash after a week, but food was enough. When it rained we slept with wet blankets. We suffered a lot because the regime entered Zambia in great numbers and attacked camps. . . . We led the life of wild animals, the situation was very bad during those times. [Musa Maphosa]

One of the guerrillas explained the difficulties the freedom fighters had in accommodating young people in their camps:

At Nampundu, there you could see human suffering. . . . There were too many to be sent for training. There were moments of real stress for many. It was the empty-handedness. At home, people had been doing things for themselves. . . . Now you could see them sitting there, soaking problems into themselves, because there was nothing to do . . . many of the schoolchildren were too small to be trained, and also by now an awareness was growing of the need for educated people in the future.

. . . We soon built up schools, without any equipment. We held classes under the trees, with blackboards on easels. After some time, there were schools in all the camps. [Comrade Matjaka]

The final excerpt touches on the poignancy of returning home in 1980 once peace had been established at Lancaster House in London:

Lancaster House conference was called. After hearing the success of the conference we jumped here and there for joy. A cease-fire was called at the same time. After the 1980 elections we returned home. We were carried by bus to Kitwe, where we boarded a train which took three days to reach Zimbabwe. We were welcomed by parents at Luveve station. Many people were surprised to see so many young people, because they believed that Ian Smith had killed all the refugees in Zambia and Mozambique. I got a warm and amazed welcome from some of my relatives. [Ngwizah Nyathi]

"THE YOUNG WHISTLING IN THE ECHOING BUSH"

Children have a talent for escaping surveillance.[6] They can move through the countryside undetected and thus serve admirably as messengers in times of war. Boys and girls aged between ten and sixteen who served the comrades were called *mujibha* and *chimbwido*, respectively. These children acquired positions of power in their communities because of their important and often dangerous roles. They were viewed with wonder because of their bravery and with fear because of their arbitrary power. If a *mujibha* denounced someone as a sell-out, the comrades took action that sometimes resulted in that person's death. A number of people told me that they had been threatened, frightened, even beaten as a consequence of evidence given by children either to the comrades or to the soldiers.

---

[6]The title of this section comes from Alec Pongweni's free translation of "Chirizevha Chapera" by Thomas Mapfumo and the Acid Band. The text of the song is given in appendix 3.

An estimated 50,000 young people acted as intermediaries between the comrades and the villagers during the war (Lan 1985, 125). The part played by these children was vital. The Security Forces called them "runners" or "sympathisers" and treated them almost as harshly as if they were armed insurgents.

A Rhodesian Intelligence Corps officer, Bob North, told Frederikse how good guerrilla intelligence was:

> Their bush telegraph—that word of mouth network—was by far superior to our intelligence. They knew exactly what the Security Forces were doing, virtually 24 hours a day, through their runners, the sympathisers, the *mujibas*. Those *mujibas* would give the terrs [terrorists] logistics, troop movements, troop strengths, and that was one of their greatest attributes as far as intelligence was concerned. [Frederikse 1982, 60]

A former *mujibha* described his actions in the war:

> Every schoolboy around here was working as a *mujiba,* when he went home after school. I just came to be a *mujiba* when the comrades first came in and told us their politics. Then we believed them. Then they began sending us to collect blankets or to look for the enemy. When I was sent to count the soldiers, I went secretly because when you are seen you are shot, of course. You look to see how many they are and what type of guns they have. You must go secretly—if you are noticed, then you are done for. [ibid.]

No doubt young people sometimes abused their positions of power. Ranger found that in Makoni in early 1981, "there was a good deal of remembered resentment among elders and parents directed against the power exercised by the *mujibhas* during the war" (1985, 292). He quotes an informant as saying "most of the people who are said to have been killed by the guerrillas are the direct victims of the *mujibhas.* These sometimes robbed civilians, abused the populace at beer parties and, in most cases, misrepresented the comrades' aims and commitments" (ibid.). Teenage girls acting as informants and messengers for the guerrillas "were able to exercise a good deal of power, for the first time in Makoni's history" (ibid., 207).

Girls were also used to serve the guerrillas in the ways that females are in wars—to cook for them, sleep with them, and gather information by making love to enemy soldiers (see the quotation from a ZANLA political commissar in Frederikse 1982, 70; see also Ranger 1985, 292). In 1980, after Independence, *mujibhas* were quickly divested of their power.

The experiences of these young people during the war—their acquisition of power and their subsequent loss of it—must have had a profound impact on their feelings of identity and their view of their position in society. During the war there was no safety for the innocent, nor were many children allowed to remain innocent. Akson Bare, a student from Chibi, told Frederikse: "We *mujibas*, we did not have any guns. Sometimes I wished I had a gun but the comrades did not trust all of us, even, though they trusted some of us. They could not just give the gun because it wanted courage, you see. If you are not courageous you cannot be given a gun because when the enemy comes you will leave the gun and run away. Then the gun will be taken by the enemy and that is a disadvantage to the comrades" (1982, 69–70).

As communities began realigning power structures after the war, children were firmly placed back into the niche of childhood. Some children acknowledged the aftereffects of trauma and sought various means of recovery. Others carried their pain silently. One young woman took ten years before she could talk of the six weeks she spent in prison. She was eleven years old when soldiers interrogated her as to the whereabouts of her sister, a *chimbwido*. She was devastated by the experience but told no one. She expressed her distress in a long series of health crises, which were eventually resolved by the intervention of a doctor who gave her physical and psychological attention.

THE MEANS TO HEAL

Spirit Mediums during the War

Two widely acclaimed books, Ranger (1985) and Lan (1985), deal with the role of spirit mediums during the war. Both authors grant a significant and important position to the spirit mediums in the struggle. Opposed to their view is the writing of Krige (1988), who dismisses the mediums' role as far less important than the violence used by the guerrillas to secure peasant cooperation. Lan represents one end of a continuum—the romantic view of guerrilla obedience to spirit mediums as the representatives of the ancestors. Krige represents the other—a cynical dismissal of the importance of peasant ideology and traditional religion in favor of the effective force of violence. Both, it seems to me, are too extreme.

Ranger (1985, 182) argues that the struggle for liberation was "quintessentially a peasant war" for the recovery of lost lands and the cessation of state interference in production. He understands that spirit mediums gave the guerrillas legitimacy in terms of the past and gave the peasants some way of controlling the young men with guns (ibid., 208). The mediums effectively laid down "the moral economy of the war" (ibid., 212).

Ranger quotes Amon Shonge on the relations between spirit mediums and guerrillas:

> This use of mediums was the same everywhere. The comrades had to contact a spirit medium first to introduce themselves. Then they would be told what to do. They were told which were the holy places and given some sort of byelaws to guide them. They were told that (they) must not kill innocent people. Nearly everyone then started to feel that the mediums were very important people. The mediums felt that they had been forgotten and now they were remembered. [ibid.]

A common focus on "lost lands" and a common belief in the protection of the spirits were included in a composite peasant-guerrilla ideology, Ranger believes. He cites three reasons for the effectiveness of this composite ideology. First, the relationship of the spirit mediums to Shona-speaking rural society was closely connected with the basics of the peasant economy. Second, the mediums participated in a "movement of cultural renewal" that covered at least two-thirds of Zimbabwe. And third, a strong element of pragmatism exists in the religion of spirit mediums (ibid., 213).

Spirit mediums, in Ranger's opinion, continue to be influential in postwar Zimbabwe:

They have continued to be influential because they are still playing the combination of roles which made them so important during the war. Their endorsement, which gave legitimacy to the guerrillas, now gives legitimacy to village committees. They can still speak in the voice of the ancestors in order to articulate the peasant political programme. And they remain relevant to rural production. [ibid., 339-40]

Bourdillon (1987a, 272) expresses some skepticism as to the dependence of guerrillas on spirit mediums. Among the eastern Korekore, at least, he feels that the mediums "acquired more status from the guerrillas than the guerrillas did from the mediums." In this area, the guerrillas had their legitimacy as freedom fighters, a new category of thought, and they required no legitimation in terms of the old categories.

The role of spirit mediums in the liberation war is difficult to characterize. Their impact seems to have varied from area to area, the period during the war and particular variables (including the strength of Christian following, class conflict, and lineage tensions in a region). Undoubtedly, though, spirit mediums played a significant part, either actually or symbolically, in certain areas for certain periods of the war.

I want to stress one difference between the spirit mediums discussed above and those with whom I worked. The former were usually the mediums of *mhondoro* spirits and the latter of more humble ancestral *midzimu* and healing *mashave*, although a few claimed to be possessed by *mhondoro* or rain spirits. The evidence I gathered, therefore, reflects on the experiences of a less-elevated population of mediums.

Healers in the War

Among the healers with whom I worked, I found a wide range of attitudes and sets of behavior in relation to the comrades. Some healers had little to do with the comrades, apart from paying the dues expected of every villager—gifts of money (often $10 a month), food, and clothing. Other healers attended to the specific needs of the comrades—for medicine, divination, advice, and intervention with the shades—as they were presented to them. Healers often explained to me that it was their duty to attend any patient and never to forsake another human being. The herbalist Rungodo claimed to have been *vabereki* (parents) to the comrades: he did not heal them but fed them and gave them information. The Security Forces heard of this and beat him. Rungodo responded to their demand for information about the comrades by saying, "I am old. I feed whomever asks. You, too, if you wish."

Mande, who is possessed by a *gombwe* spirit with rain-making powers, was the bravest of those who acted in accord with ethical standards that he believed were determined by the shades. His spirit, he says, abhors bloodshed (he would refuse to talk to me if I was wearing red). As a spirit medium and a village headman, Mande was frequently in contact with the comrades throughout the war years. He did not help them because he believed that his spirit hates bloodshed. He said, "The comrades were annoyed. My spirit does not allow killing and so I could give neither courage nor power to the comrades for killing." Yet he grants that the comrades could not have won the war without contact through mediums to the shades.

The Security Forces harassed him for information about the comrades. At first, they were harsh but did not beat him. He was jailed in Murehwa, however, and the soldiers threatened to shoot him. (The first sign that he was called by a spirit occurred in Mande's childhood when he refused to eat *sadza*—the porridge of ground grain that forms the staple food of the people in the region. His parents respected this taboo and fed him on rice when they could. The soldiers knew that he did not eat *sadza*.) For twenty days the soldiers gave him only *sadza* to eat. He refused it. His courage, he says, came from his spirit. Once the soldiers tried to beat him but they fought among themselves.

In 1978, the soldiers burned the line of houses that formed Mande's village to punish the people for having fed the comrades. On another occasion, three soldiers came to Mande's home and commanded him to return with them to the school where they and other soldiers were preparing an evening meal. They taunted Mande, demanding that he make rain fall. Eventually their commander made the soldiers stop their teasing and allowed Mande to return home. The soldiers camped near Nyahungwe, the rock mountain that is sacred in the area and that Mande climbs when he is possessed. That night, heavy rain fell and the camp was deluged. The next morning the soldiers returned to Mande to apologize.

Chidakwa, too, attempts to live in accord with ethical principles that he claims have been laid down by the shades. He says:

> A *n'anga* is like a priest: he is there to help and bring back health and well-being and not to destroy. If I should touch anything with the intention of killing or causing harm, I myself would die. Even during war, *n'anga* must protect, not destroy. Just as a sick child needs care when he wakes at night or just as children must be protected from contagious disease, so comrades needed protection.

Until 1978 Machena had little involvement with the war. One evening, early in that year, soldiers in an army vehicle arrived in his village. Machena took refuge in a room with his father-in-law and sister-in-law. They heard shots. Later they were told that the visit was a reprisal for the killing of two soldiers by the comrades. People were searched; some escaped into the hills, but others were arrested. Once the soldiers had left, rumors about sell-outs were passed around the village. Machena heard his name mentioned. A comrade visited him and asked if all was well. Machena said yes, but the comrade responded, "No. Have you heard of soldiers in the area?" He left. The next day a *mujibha*, a young messenger from the comrades, came and told Machena to follow him. He was led to the comrades' base in the mountains. On his arrival, a comrade called him a soldier and he knew that he had been identified as a sell-out. The comrades questioned him, taunted him, poked him, and took turns beating him. One man swung at him with his gun but the gun flew from his hands and landed outside the room. The comrades believed Machena was possessed and they clapped their hands to ask the spirit for forgiveness. Had he been a sell-out, Machena explained, the spirit would not have possessed him because the shades supported the fight for liberation. The comrades asked Machena for snuff, a signal that he forgave them. He was angry and sore, and so he refused. However, they had seen the snuff container hanging around his neck and helped themselves. Machena was allowed to return home. Later, the comrades lectured the villagers on not naming people as sell-outs without first carefully establishing the truth of the accusation. Machena treated his wounds with snuff. After that, he was sometimes called out by the comrades to treat or divine for them.

Masango, too, was accused of being a sell-out, but by the Security Forces, not the comrades. He had, he says, served the comrades, giving them money, food, and clothing and going out to treat them when he was called. Twice he was arrested by the soldiers. He was taken to prison, beaten, and given electric shocks. In 1982 he claimed to know the two young boys who informed on him. He has not accused them, but suspects that they suffer knowing that they did wrong and should not have yielded to a bribe. They cannot rid themselves of their suffering unless the problem is made public. That is unlikely to occur unless mental confusion assails one of them.

Some healers served the comrades often throughout the years of warfare. Chihata and Jana, for example, were frequently called out at night and they would walk for kilometers through the bush and ford rivers to attend comrades hiding in the hills. They interpreted comrades' dreams, divined for them, treated the sick, and gave information about Security Force movements. Unquestionably they were in danger and their attentions were both important and valued. Both Chihata and Jana are elderly and frail: their night ministrations could not have been easy for them.

After the war, new lines of authority were being drawn up and tested when a neighbor of Chihata's, who proclaimed himself a watchman of the ruling party's interests, persecuted her and her family; party members controlled his excesses but not his minor harassment. In 1982 former comrades were still consulted on many community issues. For example, the healers sought the comrades' permission to work with me. One healer told me that she should not keep anything from me because the comrades said I was one source through whom government could be informed about the situation in the countryside.

Facing Evil after the War

N'anga said that after the war there was more madness than before. Many spirits of people who had not been given correct ritual burials or whose deaths resulted from acts of wrongdoing remained unsettled. They said that war had retarded the thinking of children and had caused many to behave oddly.

During the war, freedom fighters invoked their spiritual links to the shades through spirit mediums, the religious representatives of the people (see Lan 1985). Having established these links, the guerrillas asserted their rights to stamp out witchcraft. Witches rend communities apart, encourage distrust and disruption, and undermine the united front necessary for fighting a guerrilla war. Claiming to have medicines that enabled them to "see" witches, the comrades killed those they identified.

Gushongo said that while the comrades had done society a service in ridding it of witches, they had not killed witches' familiars. After the war these creatures roamed the countryside stirring up evil, and it fell to ritual specialists to kill them or neutralize their powers. The spirits of those wrongfully killed as witches were said also to be returning to seek retribution.

Rituals of Expurgation

On returning from the war, men and women who had fought on either side visited healers to be cleansed. This was an important catharsis for both individuals and communities. Cleansing and protection were within the set of ritual actions in which children's distress was acknowledged and handled.

Cleansing is conducted by *n'anga* for young and old. It is an integral part of treating many illnesses and preparing for any major ritual. *N'anga* say that evil from without is being chased away and that it is not the conscience that is being cleansed. One can be cleansed of evil airs, the evil imprint from contact with a corpse, evil spirits (alien or witch), and evil actions that result from another's envy, jealousy, or ill will. Unless the patient reveals the truth, cleansing will be ineffective. And unless compensation is paid for harm caused in serious cases such as murder, trouble will continue to afflict the family, and recovery will not follow.

A patient is cleansed internally and externally. A wide range of plants (especially aromatic herbs) and animal parts are used as emetics and purgatives, through incisions in the skin, or in bathing and drinking water. *N'anga* also cleanse those to whom they teach herbal remedies or dream interpretation or whose spirits are being called out.

Babies too are cleansed. Soon after birth, a baby should be protected against illness that might be related to the fontanelle. During this treatment, the baby is usually cleansed with water in which a cowrie shell has been soaked. A baby with diarrhea may be cleansed internally with, often enough, disastrous results. In one case, the *n'anga* divined that the baby's diarrhea was caused by evil directed at her by a neighbor's jealousy of the mother's successful farming. He threw his *hakata* to determine whether or not the baby should be taken to hospital.

Cleansing is seen to strengthen the mind, chase evil, and secure protection. I could find no parallel among the Zezuru for the concept found elsewhere in Africa of cleansing as a way to clear the heart of anger (see, for example, Harris 1978). Despite suggestions from me, no *n'anga* saw the act of cleansing as a means to ease the conscience or as an opportunity to "speak out" the ill will in one's heart. Indeed, they said that the motives of one who speaks too easily in such a vein would be suspect. Most see anger in the heart as being a private matter. Even so, cleansing does clear the air, allowing normal relationships to be resumed.

After the war, Mande cleansed many children and adults. The cleansing ritual varies, depending on his spirit's response to each case. Generally, cleansing takes the following form: A patient seeking treatment contacts Mande's son, who arranges a time for consultation. The patient arrives with his or her kin or other relatives. They sit before Mande, and Mande's son plays the *mbira* to call the spirit (Mande's third son's wife and the young female relative who looks after him can also invoke the spirit without playing the *mbira*). When Mande is possessed, his spirit diagnoses the trouble and prescribes treatment. The patient is cleansed with snuff and water. Should the patient be possessed by a *ngozi,* perhaps the spirit of one wrongfully killed during the war, he or she must stay with Mande for at least a week. Mande says, "The quantity of evil committed does not matter— an evildoer can always be cleansed." He grants, however, that someone in a state of uncontrolled behavior, called *kupanduka,* may be cleansed but his or her evil actions cannot be stopped.

Mande also performed rituals to settle the spirits of those presumed dead. In this ritual, kin come to him with a goat to sacrifice. The head and hind legs of the goat are cut off, tied into a blanket, and buried: this is called *kuwunzwa* (the suffix *-unza* means "to bring"). A *sahwira* ("ritual friend") should lead the occasion.

Usilinga is another healer who lived in the Musami area. His method of treatment is different from Mande's. When patients arrive, Usilinga does not ask for details of their trouble or illness but throws the *hakata* and divines the reason for the visit. Four "bones" in particular tell him if the patient's distress is related to the shedding of blood. The left hind ankle bone of a *hwiribidi* ("antbear")—a black bone bound with two silver rings, each about one centimeter wide—points out *munyama* ("misfortune"). A white knuckle bone of a goat, again from the ankle of the left hind leg, shows if the patient is ill because he or she touched a dying person or stood on the spot where a dead person had lain. In this case, the evil contracted is not intended by the dead or dying but may be caused by contact with them. The third bone is from the right knee of a lion. Usilinga inherited this bone from his father. It too is surrounded by a silver band on which a pattern of dots has been marked. Should this bone point to the goat bone, it would denote that an alien spirit is trying to possess the patient. The fourth bone is the beak of a kingfisher and it reveals the seriousness of the illness. If the first, third, and fourth bones point to the second, for example, then the illness is one that requires the propitiation of ancestors before it can be cured.

Once he has thrown the bones, Usilinga asks the patient to describe his or her symptoms. He also checks the patient's face for signs of illness, strain, or anxiety. Fear, he says, shows especially in the face of a child. For a child to reject his or her mother and stand alone is a sign of the influence of evil. To check his findings, Usilinga throws certain *hakata*. For example, to see if a fearful child is being troubled by evil he will throw white shells and seeds of the *mungomo* tree (*Ricinodendron rautanenii,* wild almond).

One morning in July 1982, the healer's family and I watched three soldiers in full army dress arrive at Usilinga's home to be cleansed.

Each was being troubled in some way. Divination by throwing of the *hakata* revealed that the cause of the soldiers' troubles lay in their wartime experiences. Each was advised to undergo a cleansing ritual. After the divination, they were given emetics and sent into the bush for a few hours. On their return, they were given medicine to drink and told to return that evening with small bottles into which *mushonga* ("medicine") would be poured. The cleansing process took three days.

A third example of ritual cleansing comes from a healer named Gororo. A male patient was brought to her because he was disturbed and spoke nonsense. Gororo became possessed and instructed her acolyte to make an infusion of herbs and incense over which the patient had to lean covered with a blanket. After some time, he called out that he was ready to talk. He admitted to killing nine people in the war as a fighter against the Rhodesian Army. Some he killed in battle and their spirits would not return to trouble him; some he killed as *varoyi* (witches) because he believed they had eaten the corpses of comrades killed in battle; and others he killed for being sell-outs. Gororo divined that two spirits of the last category had returned to trouble him as they had been wrongfully accused. Had they been guilty, they would not have sought revenge. Gororo then cleansed the patient. The purification ritual would not have been effective if the patient had not revealed the truth.

Gushongo, a *n'anga* with a large following in Mabvuku, did not claim to have played much of a role during the war; but he has handled a great many patients whose troubles stem from those years. He gave me the names of seventeen university students (five of whom were women), who were troubled by *ngozi* as a consequence of their wartime activities.

Students and scholars troubled by *ngozi* are given medicine to hold the spirit at bay and allow them to continue their studies. Gushongo said that he has many patients at one of the top mission schools. He holds that the only way to rid a person of *ngozi* attacks is to pay compensation. He says he gives certain medicine to a family head who can administer it to close kin. If one of them should be killed unfairly, his or her spirit will trouble the murderer or witch within a week. Without this medicine it may be twenty years before the spirit may retaliate. In September 1983, Gushongo treated a patient troubled by a *ngozi.* The death had occurred during the war. The spirit of the dead person was invoked at a *bira* (ritual feast) and agreed to stop troubling the family on being told that compensation had been paid—ten cows and a young girl. Gushongo said that many girls had been given in compensation, usually girls old enough to be able to conceive.

Kazembe professes to know of four cases in which a girl was given in compensation. He said that the girl should grow up in the stranger's family, eventually have a child and, if the baby is the same sex as the family member killed, her duty will have been fulfilled. She could then marry into the family with full *roora* ("bridewealth") being paid or return home, leaving the child behind. Sometimes the gift of a girl was purely a ritual gesture. It was said that with payment of compensation, old scores were settled and the possibility for the renewal of cordial relations between families was created. If a girl refuses to go, she risks having members of her family killed off one by one. When a girl conceives, a cow is paid to her mother to prevent her *mudzimu* from causing friction by asking, Why is my child used to compensate for something she has not done?

Ritual measures to protect one's person or property usually follow cleansing. Certain categories of people are seen to be particularly vulnerable and, therefore, to need careful protection. Those include women attempting to conceive or who are pregnant, children (especially infants), people who hold positions of high rank or who are wealthy or powerful, *n'anga,* and foreigners. Protection is sought for a wide range of eventualities among which are: protection against bullets in war, against theft, against the intrusion of witches into a home, against trouble on a journey, and against others' jealousy.

Assuaging Children's Trauma

Children gain access to the care and attention of *n'anga* through illness, expression of distress, the telling of dreams (especially troubling ones), and bad behavior. Parents or other kin, having exhausted the family's means to cure or comfort, take the child to a healer. In the years immediately after the end of the war, healers were sensitive to the possibility that children had been disturbed by the conflict and might have participated in it.

When a patient presents a complex problem, whether the patient is an adult or child, the *n'anga* follows the same process. Initially the patient or a member of his or her family describes the symptoms, often in general terms to test the healer's competence to divine the trouble accurately. The *n'anga* then takes ritual steps such as throwing *hakata*, becoming possessed, or consulting the shades in some other way. He or she then describes the trouble (sometimes while possessed) and gradually explores the likely causes. Once those are agreed upon and the *n'anga* is satisfied that the patient has spoken out fully and truthfully, treatment is prescribed. (Ascertaining the truthfulness of the patient often takes time and may involve propitiating the shades during rituals when the spirits harassing the patient are called out.) If it is divined that the trouble is being caused by a *ngozi* (an aggrieved spirit) seeking compensation, then discussion may have to be arranged between family groups to resolve old quarrels. Finally, the patient is cleansed (the means used are various) and protected against future harm. Anybody has access to this ritual process of mediation among kin and family groups.

All *n'anga* I spoke to agreed that the war had disturbed children. They identified three main causes. One was that children witnessed the bloodshed and death. Gushongo said that even if a child only witnessed a killing, the *ngozi* (the unsettled spirit of the one killed) might return to trouble the child, causing him or her to relive the visions, and saying, "You were there, too." Evil must then be blocked and the cause explained to the parents. Medicine is given to the child to stop him or her reliving the experience. These cases, healers say, are the easiest to treat.

Another cause of distress was from *ngozi* seeking to revenge wrongful deaths. *Ngozi* often attacked children because they were vulnerable and precious family members. In such cases the child is a pawn. His or her well-being depends on the ability of a *n'anga* to reveal the true cause of the child's trouble and on the willingness of the family to tell the truth, pay compensation, or chase the *ngozi* to the killer.

The third cause lay in children's wartime activities. We have seen that as *mujibha* children held power over others' lives. The world turned upside down: a child could cause an adult's death. After the war, children had to live with their consciences; they had to resume positions in the community, which once more placed them near the bottom of the hierarchies defined by family, community, and school. No doubt some children knew a lot about adults' behavior during the war, and that knowledge may have been a burden during the process of realignment of power between families. I shall give one case to illustrate each of these broad sets of causes.

A boy of six was brought by his parents to Machena because he was acting strangely. He would scream, "My gun, my gun. The soldiers are here." Cleansing medicine was placed in incisions in his skin and his parents were advised to keep him under close surveillance. They were instructed not to be harsh with him, nor to shout at him, and they were told to set him small tasks and observe how he handled them. The parents were to report his progress to the *n'anga*. When his behavior had improved, he was returned to the *n'anga* so that he could be protected against further influence from evil spirits. During the treatment sessions no one was blamed for the child's odd behavior and the child was not labeled as deviant. Ritual attention and gentle care probably helped to exorcise the effects of his experience during the war.

The next two cases were handled by Gororo. In September 1982 I attended a *bira* at Gororo's home during which a girl, troubled by a *ngozi,* was treated. The girl was accompanied by a female relative and a brother-in-law from Rusape. Upon arrival at Gororo's home, they announced that she was ill; nothing was explained. That evening, Gororo was possessed at the *bira.* She divined that a kinsman of the girl had murdered (*umhondi*) someone during the war. The patient and her relatives said, "We heard about that." (Gororo pointed out that one never admits to knowledge of a crime thus exposed but only agrees to having heard of it.)

During the *bira,* the *ngozi* spoke through the girl asking, "Are you trying to kill me again?" The spirit called for five cattle to be paid in compensation. The patient was then treated with aromatic herbs. The healer warned that the girl's illness would continue if the truth had been withheld or if compensation was not paid. Sometimes the *ngozi* can be "chased" to another family member more closely related to the murderer or to the murderer, if he or she is alive. The spirit will give clues as to who the murderer is, and family discussions should reveal the culprit.

When I suggested that revenge taken in this form is hard on the innocent, especially children, Gororo said, "There is no way to avoid it. It is part of the system."

Immediately after the war Gororo treated many cases of young boys with guilty consciences (*zviito zvavakaita*). Each was closely questioned by Gororo's spirit. Some were found to have caused people to die but to have had no choice given the conditions of war. Yet, some still felt guilty, the spirit revealed. The boys were cleansed and given medicine to prevent them from reliving their experiences. Gororo warned them that those who lied about their experiences during the war would find no relief. Gororo's spirit identified one boy as having lied. The spirit said that during the war he had hit a neighbor on the head and that person had subsequently died: now a *ngozi* was troubling members of the boy's family.

The third case involved a sixteen-year-old girl who was brought by her mother from Bulawayo to see Chihata in Musami. The girl had fought in the war and since her return had been acting oddly. She had been singing war songs, beating her mother, saying, "I want my money," and acting childishly. She was given a purgative, and medicine was rubbed into incisions in her skin and placed in her drinking water. It was divined that a *ngozi* was affecting her. Apparently another *n'anga* had divined the same cause and her family had paid compensation to the family of the person whose death the girl had caused. But the girl still needed treatment, according to the Musami *n'anga*. The girl was possibly, in part, rebelling against her return to the conservative norms and forms of control of her family. Unfortunately I do not know whether the traditional form of resolution offered her any comfort.

Rituals of purification helped eliminate some of the defilement of war. Wrongs were straightened out through confession and sometimes compensation. As hosts of the shades, healers have access to privileged knowledge about the thoughts and past deeds of their patients. They examine motives and intention in order to straighten out mystical disorder.

Taussig scorns anthropologists for having "bound the concept of ritual hand and foot to the imagery of order, to such an extent that order is identified with the sacred itself, thereby casting disorder into the pit of evil" (1987, 444). Perhaps we need to stress that the possibility exists for ritual specialists to create order and stir disorder. For example, Bourdillon emphasizes that "spirit mediums have a degree of independence from all political controls, and this independence suited them to the role of disturbing the existing order and the existing political control in the 1970s [i.e., during the War of Liberation]," (1984-85, 48). An alternative, more destructive attempt to purify the community and measures taken to limit the damage are illustrated by appendix 10.

CONCLUSION

Healers played a profound role in the reordering of Zimbabwean society after the war. In responding to post-war conditions they were creative, flexible, and caring in a way that demonstrates their integrity within communities.

Children suffered during the war and displayed their distress after the war. Their unhappiness or ill health was channeled into existing means for addressing distress. Healers responded to their need by mediating between the shades and the community on behalf of the individual. They gave ritual attention (often in the form of rituals to cleanse and protect) and personal care, they listened and probed for the truth, and they monitored responses over time. Healers could attend to stress expressed by members of communities and as evidenced in individual behavior because they are members of those communities. Healers were sensitive to individual and community needs because they too experienced war and observed the range of response, activity, and emotional play that war calls forth. Also they are the guardians of ritual (though they hold no monopoly and are constantly informed and directed in their ritual performance by kin, neighbors, and fellow *n'anga*). Healers take advantage of the flexibility and elasticity that informs Zezuru interpretation of spiritual affairs. Zezuru cosmology is not hamstrung by theory that divides body from mind. Consequently, a child's (or an adult's) need for healing—displayed in physical, mental, or spiritual terms—will be taken seriously, leading to divination and ritual care and attention. Whatever the nature of a child's problem, he or she can claim the attention of society's specialists and can be directly involved in society's ritual means of curing, explaining, and comforting.

My intention is not to romanticize the role of healers; I do not claim that they necessarily succeed in their attempts to heal. They may, in certain circumstances, represent the forces of convention in constricting individual freedom and they may abuse the trust placed in them by patients. But those caveats can be made in relation to healers in any system; some are more adept at fielding blame and disguising control than others. I was deeply impressed by the commitment and concern of healers in their handling of troubled children.

CHAPTER FOUR

ZEZURU TURN OF THE SCREW: ON CHILDREN'S EXPOSURE TO EVIL

INTRODUCTION

THE THEME of this chapter is the *exposure* of children to evil.[1] I want to explore Zezuru notions of the innocence of children: their vulnerability to evil; their access to the supernatural; their complicity in evildoing; their ability to judge and bring retribution for evil done; and their need for protection and cleansing. Each of these issues arises in the novella by Henry James *The Turn of the Screw*. I use this story to frame my exploration of Zezuru notions of evil and childhood for several reasons.

First, for fun: certainly mine and, perhaps, yours. Second, because I want to use James's story to recreate the atmosphere of fear that accompanies the possibility of possession by demons. Many of us trained

---

[1]Hannan (1984) gives the following translations from English to Shona:

evil [adj.]: *muvi* [n.]: *uipi;* evil-doer: *munyangadzi;* one suspected of being an eil-doer: *garan'anga;* evil done in return for good: *jida;* evil purpose: *hwoni;* to wish evil to [verb, transitive]: *nangaidza.*

bad (morally) [adj.]: *muvi;* bad (morally) person: *muipi;* to become bad (morally): *nyangara;* person who is a bad influence on others: *makonyonga.*

in the so-called rational system of Western scientific education have little experience of fear that derives from supernatural evil and danger. (We have, of course, an abundance of other fears and face evil in many guises.) Pocock, surveying British uses of the term *evil,* finds two points of view: "A majority is prepared to use the word in the radical sense of inhumanly monstrous, and so to engage in an absolute distinction between acceptable and unacceptable kinds of human being. A minority is reluctant to use the word at all, because, Pocock suggests, it is too strong and reveals a reluctance to so totally convert fellow humans into monsters" (Parkin 1985, 12–13). Contrary to Pocock, Macfarlane claims that the word *evil* is now used in its weak sense, "meaning to cause discomfort and/or pain, to be unpleasant, offensive and disagreeable, to be 'not good.' It is interchangeable with 'bad,' 'unpleasant,' 'harmful.'" He adds, "The disappearance of evil as a concept is one of the most extraordinary features of modern society. That it is no longer generally possible to conceive of an abstract force of evil is clearly of great interest to historians and anthropologists" (1985, 57). My third reason for drawing on the story is that James has brilliantly crystallized each turn of the screw that sets evil into the experience of childhood. It is a parable on the irrationality of fear. The story's effect relies on shared notions of evil and, as I discovered while seeking to trace the transmission of knowledge from traditional healers to following generations, those notions are pooled and passed on. A commonly held belief in the sources of evil—in the characterization of what is natural or unnatural, in the means to ward off evil, and in the nature of destiny, damnation, or doom—underlies the identification of cause in illness or trouble. The identification in turn directs treatment and protection.

In trying to unravel how childhood is conceived, I soon realized that these conceptions are reflected in the perceived relationship between evil, illness, death, and treatment. Perhaps others will be encouraged to compile an indigenous psychology. I did not set out to study the phenomenology of evil. Nor is there any published writing on its place in Zezuru cosmology. The topic was forced on my attention during research on healers and childhood. James's story provoked me into focusing, while analyzing my data, on certain aspects of the relation between notions of evil and healing.

Just as James uses the theme of possession of children to raise questions about the phenomena of evil, so a study of childhood concepts led me to consider Zezuru notions of evil. This confirms a point of methodology that deserves wider attention—the study of children necessitates reflection on the beliefs and practices current within society and examination of the interchange between children and adults as they shape those beliefs.

This chapter examines in three sections the exposure of children to evil: innocence, identity, and evil. Each section is preceded by a selection from *The Turn of the Screw*. A summary of the chapter's themes follows.

For Zezuru, children are pure: they represent nonevil. They belong to the shades. Their innocence does not imply a state of passivity. Rather, children's own resources are bolstered by the protection afforded by living and dead kin. This is different from a notion of children as innocents who are corruptible and therefore in need of control (see Swartz and Levett 1990, for a discussion of that view). Children are from an early age seen to be responsible for their actions. Children's innocence or purity is mirrored in the concept of adult purity. For example, the search for knowledge requires purity. Ethical issues to do with morality and responsibility shape ideals of adult purity. The converse is madness or evil. And these are based in a failure of identity, of the integrity of self.

To be secure in identity is to possess an integrity of self that guards against vulnerability. (To be vulnerable is to be innocent, without defenses and without the need to retaliate.) Children's identity is initially marked by the giving of names. Identity is formed in relation to an individual's position in the family, community, and the world of the spirits. Children are active in shaping their ascribed positions, forming identities for themselves that may even redefine others' perceptions of their assigned places within communities. Identity is socially constructed: a person cannot act alone. The establishment and maintenance of good relations with kin and ancestors are a necessity. Possession by evil spirits is a replacement of self by other.

This leads into the problem of what is evil. In the third section of this chapter, I consider ambiguity and the pooled imaginings of terror, jealousy, and envy in relation to Henry James's story. These are related to children's knowledge of adult evil and therapy. Sources of misfortune are outlined and the notion of ancestors as conscience or superego is pondered. In the examination of evil as witchcraft, children are seen as caught in the midst of the battle between good and evil. Zezuru links between witches and spirits are drawn. Spirits can kill and, we learn, there are ways to kill witches.

The conflict between parents and children is an expression of evil. Society has formulated ways to control the conflict and limit its possible harm. Finally, the knowledge of evil is used as social control; the knowledge is latent or dormant most of the time.

Evil Possession of a Young Girl

Before giving an outline of the novella by Henry James I shall briefly describe a case of evil possession of a young girl that happened in Musami not long before I worked there. It shows that witchcraft is seen as utterly evil, a threat to vitality and life force and a source of the uncanny. It takes little imagination to recreate the awfulness of the woman's end and the girl's madness. During Zimbabwe's War of Liberation the guerrilla fighters tackled the sources of witchcraft wherever they identified them. The guerrillas claimed to be guided by the shades in "smelling out" evil. Just before the end of the war, guerrillas sought to eradicate witchcraft in a home in Musami.

The mother-in-law of an important village headman wore a white belt around her waist in which was wrapped a charm, a *zango*. Towards the end of Zimbabwe's War of Liberation some members of the guerrilla forces saw the belt and, using special powers said to derive from the spirits, "knew" that it was really a snake belonging to a witch spirit that possessed the old woman. They burned the belt and the woman lay down and died. Her life was in the belt of witchcraft. Shortly after that, her eighteen-year-old granddaughter left home. She moved about telling the spirits who she was, but they ignored her and she disappeared. She has never been seen again. It is said that when she was fifteen her grandmother had initiated her into witchcraft, passing on a *shave* to her. The family was powerful in the area, and other tales of witchcraft were rumored about them.

A Tale of Possession

The Turn of the Screw is a masterpiece of its kind—a powerful tale of "possession" as in the old fables of demons and dybbuks. The story purports to come from a manuscript written by a young governess whose part in the tale is central. The governess (she is given no name in the story) applies for a position caring for two orphaned children in a country manor. She is young and inexperienced and has come straight from her clergyman father's home. She is interviewed by the children's uncle and accepts the post despite his injunction that she should never trouble him—neither appeal to nor complain nor write about anything; only meet all questions herself, receive all moneys from his solicitor, take the whole thing over and let him alone.

The governess travels to the manor, meeting first eight-year-old Flora then ten-year-old Miles. Both children enchant her with their fairytale beauty, innocence, freshness, and purity. Soon her contentment is shattered when she sees the ghosts of Peter Quint and Miss Jessel, former employees at the manor. The governess "feels" that they have come to draw the children away into danger. She becomes obsessed and sets herself up as their "shield," serving as an "expiatory victim."

An atmosphere of evil is cleverly built up. Through the eyes of the governess we watch the threat to the children grow. Many critics, including Leon Edel (1971), hold that the evil is in her own mind. Her circumstantial account of the behavior of the children establishes them as "normal." Yet the governess makes them seem sinister. The real "turn of the screw"—the particular twist of pain in the tale—resides in what the governess is doing to the children. They, on their side, try constantly to accommodate themselves to her vision. In the end, the girl flees from the governess in the care of the housekeeper. But the boy dies in her arms. Were the children possessed? Were they in danger from the former servants? Were they in complicity with evil? Was the governess foolish, romantic, hysterical, and neurotic? Was there a fight for the possession of innocent children? What is the source of the evil air that permeates the tale?

The story originated in a tale recalled by the archbishop of Canterbury on the evening of January 10, 1895, as he and Henry James told ghost stories round the fire. James recorded it in his notebook on January 12, 1895:

> Note here the ghost-story told me at Addington (evening of Thursday 10th), by the Archbishop of Canterbury: the mere vague, undetailed, faint sketch of it—being all he had been told (very badly and imperfectly), by a lady who had no art of relation, and no clearness: the story of the young children (indefinite number and age) left to the care of servants in an old country-house, through the death, presumably, of parents. The servants, wicked and depraved, corrupt and deprave the children; the children are bad, full of evil, to a sinister degree. The servants *die* (the story is vague about the way of it) and their apparitions, figures, return to haunt the house *and* children, to whom they seem to beckon, whom they invite and solicit, from across dangerous places, the deep ditch of a sunk fence, etc.—so that the children may destroy themselves, lose themselves, by responding, by getting into their power. So long as the children are kept from them, they are not lost; but they try and try and try, these evil presences, to get hold of them. It is a question of the children "coming over to where they are." It is all obscure and imperfect, the picture, the story, but there is a suggestion of strangely gruesome effect in it. The story to be told—tolerably obviously—by an outside spectator, observer. (James, quoted in Edel 1971, 425-26; emphasis in original).

James read the note eighteen months later and made of it a "fantastic fiction." He is quoted as saying, "I meant to scare the whole world with that story." He made it a story of "belief" and "allegation": the belief is centered in the mind of one person, the narrator, who is the children's governess. "The story told is strange, filled with terror and passion; and so arranged that we must decide for ourselves the credibility of the witness. It is on this question that the countless interpretations of this tale have hinged" (Edel 1971, 427)[b]. In writing the tale, James delved into the "deep well of unconscious cerebration" and drew on the "queer dim play of consciousness" (James, quoted in ibid., 429). James wrote of the story that he wanted to create the impression of "the communication to the children of the most infernal imaginable evil and danger—the condition on their part of being as exposed as we can humanly conceive children to be" (letter to F. W. H. Myers; quoted by Edel, 429; emphasis in the original). And that is the theme that threads through the present chapter.

INNOCENCE

The children, Miles and Flora, are presented through their governess's eyes as, initially at least, innocent. Flora is described as "one of Raphael's holy infants" (445); she has a "fathomless charity" (479); a "blest innocence" and a "bloom of health and happiness" (453). Miles has a "glow of freshness" and a "fragrance of purity"; he is "divine" (452) and there is a "rose-flush" to his innocence (459); he is "an angel" (459) and "too fine and fair" for school (459); he is a "little fairy prince" (496). Once the governess sniffs evil in the air she declares the children "blameless and foredoomed" (484) and sets out to protect their innocence: "I was there to protect and defend the little creatures in the world the most bereaved and the most loveable, the appeal of whose helplessness had suddenly become only too explicit, a deep constant ache of one's own engaged affection" (471).

The place Zezuru assign children in the cosmological whole is paradoxical. On the one hand, a child is a gift from the shades and must be cherished as such or retribution from the shades may swiftly follow. On the other hand, shades have no compunction about creating distress, illness, or even death for a child in the cause of maintaining order between the world of the spirits and the living, among kin and within communities. These attitudes have important implications for the care of children. Neglect or abuse of a child may set off reverberations that stir the anger of the spirits. Yet a child's illness may have to be seen within the context of social and religious relations over which the parent or caretaker may have little control.

Inherent in an adult's care of a child is the possibility that he or she may harm the child by virtue of unethical, immoral, or irresponsible behavior. For example, a woman in difficult labor may be forced to confess past adulteries to unblock the passage for the baby's birth (see Berglund 1989). A second example is the fear adults have of traveling with an infant, as measures taken to prevent harm from affecting the infant may not be powerful enough against the general ill will that strangers, whose moral worth one cannot estimate, may project.

Let us see how the Zezuru pair innocence and evil. Zezuru acknowledge three types of supernatural evil: one that is inherited, one that is transmitted through alien spirits, and another through aggrieved spirits. If the spirit of a witch can be inherited, can babies be born evil? Can children be described as witches? Can children practice witchcraft? Can they be possessed without knowing it by spirits whose intentions are bad? How can one tell the difference between plain bad behavior and badness derived from supernatural sources?

N'anga claim that a baby is always born innocent of evil. This is said despite their accord with the common belief that witchcraft is inherited. The inheritance seems to be latent, a potential that must be activated by some outside force—such as through the mother's initiation of the baby into evil or through possession by an evil spirit from among the baby's ancestors. A baby is protected by the shades from the very moment of its birth. Although the baby is born pure, he or she is extremely vulnerable—vulnerable before the anger of the shades and the evil of witchcraft and the mischance of natural illness. Protection from the shades is essential but not foolproof. Adults in the family must perform certain rituals, administer specific medicines, and observe taboos on behalf of the baby in order to bolster the protection and ensure its efficacy. If the baby's vulnerability is not to be exposed the family must act in accord with society's expectations of responsible and caring adults, both in relation to one another and to the spirit world.

The shades often cause illness or distress to fall on the baby because, the *n'anga* say, the family will pay immediate attention, seek out the cause, and attempt to redress grievances when a baby's wellbeing is affected. One *n'anga* said, "It takes a child to hurt relatives"; and another explained, "The anger of the shades is expressed through an innocent child because more pain is felt by the adults, who then seek the reason more actively and attend to its redress more quickly." Yet another *n'anga* said, "It is impossible for a baby to anger the shades, but the shades use the child as a weapon." In clarifying why it is that an innocent child may be made to suffer by the shades, a *n'anga* explained: "A person is a tree and can be shaken at any time. So if one makes a mistake, the shades cause problems to one's child." (For a careful look at the relationship between the shades and the living in terms of protection and retribution, see Kiernan 1982.)

The baby is at the mercy of the family. If the baby is not contented and well, adults should inspect their relationships and attend to their obligations. In doing so, they may call on a *n'anga*. Turner observed that among the Ndembu "part of the work of a doctor is to encourage people to discharge the obligations of their status well and not seek escape from them" (1967, 375). Conversely, the baby is powerful as an essential link in the kinship system that crosses over into the awesome sphere of the spirits. Even quite young children learn how to exploit this delicate balance in their own interest.

A child's innocence, however, is no protection. If there is disharmony in the family, or if ritual obligations have not been fulfilled, or if kin have behaved immorally, then the child's protective armor has weak spots and evil can enter in. Some *n'anga* deny that a child can be possessed by an evil spirit, though they admit that a child can be used for evil ends. Others say a child can be possessed and may be unconscious of it: only divination can tell.[2] A witch, for instance, may abuse her own children. She initiates them into evil, often by making them accustomed to the taste of human flesh. The child cannot practice witchcraft but is given the taste for, the feeling of, the need to pursue nefarious ends. A witch is said to select her favorite child, often an attractive, clever, good child, to initiate into her craft. An old and highly respected healer, Chihata in Musami believes that "a good child is more vulnerable to the influences of a bad mother. If one is rough, one refuses to do as bid while the good child will obey and so grow close to the mother." Witches are said to use their own children in paying for favors. One healer explained: "There is no evil in children. It comes naturally by seeing and doing evil."

---

[2]On children and witchcraft (their ability to practice it or their vulnerability to a parent's witchcraft) see Evans-Pritchard 1982, 31); Wyllie (1982, 135); Krige (1982, 266); and Demos (1982, 67, 69, 150, and 154).

The following example is one of possession by a malignant force of a twelve-year-old boy in Mabvuku:

Upon hearing that a certain healer was good at exorcizing spirits from children, the boy's parents brought him for consultation. The boy had shown signs of mental confusion for the fortnight before he was brought to the *n'anga*.

Upon arrival, the boy talked nonsense. He was divined for and it was seen that two spirits were trying to possess him. One was evil and came from his ancestral spirits of long ago. This spirit was blocking a good spirit, thus making the boy ill. The boy was cleansed of the evil spirit. He spent four days and four nights in the home of the *n'anga,* during which time he was taken to the bush and a black hen was used to exorcise the spirit. The boy's home was also cleansed. The boy's parents were instructed to ensure that he avoid eating pumpkin leaves, okra, peanuts, and cabbage. If he ate them, his spirit would "go round and round." Nor could he swim in rivers because the good spirit trying to possess him is a *njuzu* (river) spirit and might take him beneath the water. In their ignorance, the boy's parents may cry for him and thus lose him forever. The parents were told to watch his behavior and, if it was unusual, they should clap their hands as a welcome to the spirit, in case the spirit is seeking to say something. The *n'anga* did not anticipate bad behavior as now a good spirit was in charge of the boy.

The spirit is a healing one (as all *njuzu* spirits are) and will make itself known only in special situations, such as, for instance, to protect family relations if a fight breaks out. The spirit was appealed to by the healer's spirit to allow the boy to complete his education (he was in Grade Seven) before fully directing his life. Should the parents attempt to manipulate the situation (perhaps for their own ends by setting up the boy as a healer to earn money), the boy would soon become mentally confused. Treatment and cure of such a case would be difficult and would take time but could be done.

Appendix 11, an excerpt from a Zimbabwean writer's work, shows how a nightmare can be shaped around the concept of *njuzu*.

Because children are pure, they are helpful to healers in collecting herbs, preparing medicine, calling up the healers' spirits, and even treating patients. One healer encourages his child to rub medicine into incisions on patients' skin because the child's innocence of sin is a balm. Once a child begins to indulge in sex or a girl begins to menstruate, purity is lost.

N'anga make a direct link between purity and the pursuit of knowledge. No witch, they say, will maintain over time and with consistency the search for knowledge that is an adjunct to successful healing. Quacks or spirits with evil designs are exposed as they soon lose interest in the healing process. Overing (1985b), in a stimulating discussion of concepts of evil among the Piaroa of the Venezuelan rain forest, shows that they are conscious of the need to control the wildness in culture through knowledge. However, much of knowledge is poisoned by the potential for madness and evil (255), and its mastery demands the development of will and responsibility. Great wizards (diviners) continue to learn throughout their lives (270). They must cleanse themselves each night of the poisonous madness that lies within the forces of knowledge (256). Wickedness, a madness, is caused by the poison of unmastered knowledge (260). Their theory of knowledge emphasizes responsibilities:

> Social responsibility requires the knowledge of morality and social rules; while wizardly responsibility, extensive mastery over cultural knowledge, entails far more than the knowledge and the playing out of sociality. To take within oneself a large number of capabilities gives one a greater awareness of the nature of the cosmos, a knowledge of what the world is. . . . learning must always be a gradual process; to know too much is to become insane, absurd and madly foolish, a state in which one can do evil. [274]

By drawing attention to the Piaroa theory of knowledge, I want to suggest that current literature on Zezuru cosmology is woefully inadequate in its explication of links between concepts of morality, responsibility, and knowledge. We need to follow the leads that purity and innocence trace through these concepts and their contradistinction to madness and evil. Bourdillon (1987b, 178), for example, in drawing a comparison between the initiation and practice of healers and witches, takes into account neither the nature of the ethics in accord with which healers conduct their affairs (breach of which has serious spiritual and public consequences), nor their dependence on a watchful public (patients come largely in response to a system of referrals based on the healers' reputations), nor the value placed on the pursuit of knowledge.

In *The Turn of the Screw* the children are initially seen by the governess as innocent. Gradually their innocence is questioned and the possibility of their complicity with evil forces is raised. Finally they are seen to belong (or to be in danger of belonging) to the spirits.

Zezuru see children as innocent but vulnerable, even at birth, to the forces of evil. As children grow into adulthood and assume responsibility for their own moral stance they make a gradual transition from a state of purity to one of impurity. The Zezuru concept of the purity of children is complemented by their demand that certain adults achieve purity too, especially pregnant women, mothers of infants, and traditional healers. It may be said that the transition from childhood to adulthood is the transition from innocence to a social identity and an integrity of selfhood. This is explored in the next section.

IDENTITY

Part of the success of *The Turn of the Screw* relies on the sense of evil penetrating an isolated homestead. The children and their governess are virtually cut off from the rest of the world. Even once the summer ends, the boy is not sent back to school. The governess controls their communication with the world outside. The children are given no firm identity. We, of course, see them only through the eyes of the governess, who initially idealizes them and, finally, sees them as the accomplices of evil. Her egocentricity however pervades the tale. She admits to "my endless obsession" (515); she takes it upon herself to "form" Flora (445); she confesses "my ignorance, my confusion and perhaps my conceit" (453); sees the children as an "antidote to my pain" (460); notes that "levity is not our tone" (480); acknowledges the excess in her surveillance of the children— "my inexorable, my perpetual society" (505); and she feels that her "equilibrium depended on the success of my rigid will" (539). Her self-concern reaches a point of crisis when, having decided that Miles is in complicity with evil spirits, she is suddenly drawn up sharply and wonders:

> I seemed to float not into clearness, but into a darker obscure, and within a minute there had come to me out of my very pity the appalling alarm of his being perhaps innocent. It was for the instant confounding and bottomless, for if he *were* innocent, what then on earth was I? [548; emphasis in original]

Given their isolation, the children rely on the good sense and integrity of one woman, the governess. One turn of the screw in the story is that the integrity of the governess's inner state was ill formed for the task of protecting children from evil. The challenge is how to describe that integrity: the governess arrives at a position in which, to prove her credibility and her sanity, she has to establish the children's complicity with evil. Needham (1981, 66) holds that anthropologists have given too little attention to the classification of inner states, that is, indigenous psychology, and that few attempts have been made to specify the description of inner states in relation to context. One of those neglected states is the description of identity. Mauss (1985, 1, first published in 1938) called the idea of "person," of "self," "imprecise, delicate and fragile, one requiring further elaboration. . . . Each one of us finds it natural, clearly determined in the depths of his consciousness, completely furnished with the fundaments of the morality which flows from it." The challenge, for anthropologists, is how to understand and describe the category for others. For Mauss, the category has deep moral implications, and they are pertinent to our present concern.

Literature is one source in the search for description. The Zimbabwean writer Dambudzo Marechera gives a brilliant parable on the pull between a search for identity and ties to kin in his story "The Writer's Grain":

There was the story my father had told me, when I was barely six years of age, about the resilience of human roots: a youth rebelling against the things of his father had one morning fled from home and had travelled to the utmost of the earth where he was so happy that he wrote on the wall the words "I have been here" and signed his new name after the words; the years rolled by with delight until he tired of them and thought to return home and tell his father about them. But when he neared home his father, who was looking out for him, met him and said, "All this time you thought you were actually away from me, you have been right here in my palm." And the father opened his clenched hand and showed the son what was written in his hand. The words—and the very same signature—of the son were clearly written in the father's open palm: "I have been here." The son was so stunned and angry that he there and then slew his father and hung himself on a barren fig-tree which stood in the garden. [1978, 128]

To mark his rebellion and the distance he had placed between his father and himself, the son chose a new name and wrote it on the wall at "the utmost of the earth." Yet, when he returned home, his proclamation "I have been here" and his new name were written on his father's palm. La Fontaine (1985a, 132) suggests that in Western societies the conferring of a name identifies personhood and individuality from the beginning. In Africa, names are not so closely tied to identity: a person may acquire a number of names across time, even selecting his or her own name. A name may be used to mark a new status, for example, as inheritor of another's position and wealth. Favret-Saada believes that "witchcraft is spoken words; but these spoken words are power, and not knowledge or information" (1980, 9). Marachera plays with the power in words, naming, and the uncanny.

Suppose Zezuru healers were to judge the character of the governess and her suitability for her role as the guardian of children. It is as an intermediary between the living and the dead that the governess failed. Or so they might say. She was open to the supernatural world and Zezuru would find her contact with it quite understandable, though the form that her contact took (seeing apparitions) would be unusual. What Zezuru would question is the governess's assumption that she could "save or shield" (478) the children from the world of spirits. She made three basic errors. One was to set herself up as a shield between the living and the dead without investigating her own position vis-à-vis the spirits who appeared before her. When dealing with the shades it is imperative to examine one's heart in preparation for drawing the spirits out so that they may state their wishes or air their grievances. Neither step should be taken without reference to and the help from kin and established diviners. To assume the right to negotiate between the living and the dead without such preparation is to transgress and lay oneself open to charges of evil intention.

The second error committed by the governess leads from the first: she tried to handle the situation alone, isolating the children from their one kinsman and church leaders (her first transgression was to have accepted the conditions laid down by her employer—a compact with the devil?). At two crucial points in the story, she turned her back on the church and twice refused to comply with others' pleas to call in the children's uncle. She even kept the letters that the children wrote to their uncle: "They were too beautiful to be posted; I kept them myself; I have them all to this hour" (505). Zezuru would see the actions of the young woman as irresponsible because she violated the code that directs relations between ancestors and their living kin. If spirits are trying to possess children, then the problem is ipso facto one to be dealt with by kin. Given the innocence of children, it is likely that the grievances of the spirits are against kin or that the protection of the shades has been withdrawn and so senior members of the family must be consulted.

It could be, Zezuru might say, that the children's mother was a witch and had initiated them into witchcraft before she died. She is not mentioned in the text. If she was a witch and if the children are in complicity with the witch's acolytes (Peter Quint and Miss Jessell) there is all the more reason to call in kin and senior religious leaders to cleanse the children and cast out all evil.

The governess's third error lay in her excessive concern with and investment in her own feelings and needs. Her egocentricity is overwhelming and her obsession cannot but obscure, in Zezuru eyes, her role as a "pocket." She is, according to Zezuru ethics, without direction, lost without a code of behavior, and wrong in abrogating the role of the ancestors, relying rather on her own will.[3]

Zezuru would grant that the children could have been possessed or that spirits could be trying to lead them into evil ways. They would admit the possibility of the children's complicity with evil forces. What, for Zezuru, would be inexplicable is the crass way in which their governess attempted to shield and protect them. In assuming powers beyond her position, she lays herself open to charges of witchcraft.

I tie Zezuru thought to a ghost story but the points that I wish to make are important. Spirits affect the living and sometimes their desires and intentions (often capricious) need to be interpreted. *N'anga* see themselves as pockets (*homwe*) for the spirits. They are selected for their "hearts"—that is, their strength, trustworthiness, and honesty—and serve as conduits through whom the spirits reach the living. Their major concern is the maintenance of order among kin, within communities, and between the living and the dead. *N'anga* serve long apprenticeships under the direction of their possessing spirits before they are allowed to handle serious cases in which matters of order are expressed. The dedication and worth of *n'anga* are tested through dreams, personal travail, and their performances as healers and diviners. Kin and neighbors also watch, weigh, and judge the authenticity and wisdom of *n'anga*. Seldom is a serious case referred to only one diviner. Cases involving possession must finally be examined at a community ritual (*bira*) to which senior *n'anga* in the area are invited and at which the spirit(s) in question are called out before kin and neighbors. That is to say, anyone called on to treat serious cases to do with children's welfare ought to have been carefully vetted by the shades and the community before being countenanced

---

[3]Lienhardt believes that religious conviction molds ideas of the self: "how men see themselves must be influenced by how, or if, they see the gods" (1985, 153). He suggests, with particular reference to the Dinka, that the profound religious orientation of many African peoples' thought, their respect for the gods, condemns egotism and egoism.

as one fit to care for children. A code of ethics prevails among *n'anga* just as in the healing professions defined by modern science.

Among the Zezuru an adult or a child may be possessed. The possessing spirit may be evil. Evil spirits can disguise themselves, appearing initially as *midzimu* (family spirits) until they are accepted and only then showing their true colors. During possession, the self is temporarily replaced by a spirit. The person possessed has no subjective experience of possession. There is a loss, in some sense, of self-control. Personal identity is canceled or set aside or swamped during the process of direct negotiation. Does it take a person with a strong, confident sense of identity to consciously set aside self and be taken over by a spirit? Or is the opinion (often expressed in the popular press in Zimbabwe) that one who becomes possessed resembles most closely one of society's deviants—the mad, the paranoid, the illusionist, the shyster—closer to the truth? A careful study of children said to be possessed—their attitudes toward self, whether they feel that they have lost control or can manipulate kin in terms of socially expected responses, the context in which they see their situation, the roles into which they are cast, the use made of their plight—may increase our understanding significantly.

Drawing on cases in my field notes, I shall elaborate on the question of identity as represented in the role of kin in handling children who suffer under the influence of spirits. The following situations of two people were widely discussed in Musami as if they were parables (they are mirror images of Marachera's parable) warning people not to transgress ritual or action that accords with the expectations of kin:

An adolescent boy was mentally ill. Two healers in Musami were treating him. The boy, they said, was troubled by a spirit— the lost spirit of his father who had died at a place unknown to his kin and had not been settled. The boy's father was Malawian and his mother Zezuru. She took it upon herself to discard the boy's totem (inherited through his father's line) and call him by her own clan's totem. She attempted to cut his ties to his father's heritage hoping that the boy's troubles would abate. His madness intensified. The solution that both *n'anga* offered was for him to return to Malawi and perform rituals for settling his father's spirit.

This boy was often to be seen wandering through the villages. His madness—his loss of identity—was traced to the break in the chain that links him to his father and his ancestors.

I met the woman, described below, on a number of occasions. She was usually bent double scrubbing in the earth near a grave:

> People say that the woman is mad. She moves like a hare and spends her days near the graves of her husband and her son. She lives alone and neighbors care for her. A *n'anga* reported that on her husband's death she failed to take her children to live near kin but stayed on in an area where neither she nor her husband had ties. Her son died and now the ancestors trouble her asking why she did not return with her children to her natal home. People refer to her situation, warning each other of the consequences that failure to maintain family links may have: in the event of death, the woman was left alone in the world and went mad with grief.

A person's identity is closely tied to his or her position in the family, community, and the world of the spirits. Nevertheless, it is wrong to assume that the child accepts a given identity and does not take an active role in shaping it and directing kin's responses, even if recognized routes are followed.

In the last section it was suggested that the transition from childhood to adulthood is the transition from innocence to a social identity and an integrity of selfhood. Perhaps evildoers are adults who have failed to achieve that transition according to the norms and ethics of their community. The victims of evil are the innocent (children) and inadequate (adults). Healing aims to establish, reestablish, or strengthen a workable social identity and integrity of self.

EVIL

In *The Turn of the Screw* there is no doubt that evil is abroad, if only in the hysterical imaginings of the young governess. In conjuring up a ghostly atmosphere, Henry James imitated the gloom that the Brontës so effectively evoked in their novels and he hinted at the witch trials of earlier European and American experience. He uses ambiguity to create so effectively a sense of evil. He has the governess write, "Nothing was more natural than that these things should be the other things they absolutely were not" (473).

In explaining his technique, James said, "So long as the events are veiled, the imagination will run riot and depict all sorts of horrors. . . ." (quoted in Edel 1971, xii). In his preface, written ten years after publishing the story, James told how he had set the scene for the reader to draw on his own store of horror: "Only make the reader's general vision of evil intense enough . . . and his own experience, his own imagination . . . will supply him quite sufficiently with all the particulars. Make him think the evil, make him think it for himself, and you are released from weak specifications" (ibid.).

The Zezuru concept of evil similarly relies on a general vision of evil and the pooled imaginings of individuals. What James creates for us is an atmosphere of extrahuman evil in an ordinary setting—"The terror of the usual" (Edel 1971, ix). It is into this atmosphere that Zezuru can slip, drawing upon their shared notions of the nature of evil.

Bear in mind that while I sat and talked with *n'anga* or watched them divine, treat patients, collect and prepare medicines, discuss cases, and conduct rituals, children were almost always there—watching, listening, and sometimes participating. Children are aware of their elders' ideas of the canker of evil and they collect their own stock of lore about evil. One child solemnly warned me, "If you whistle at night you may be bewitched." I overheard two other children (the grandchildren of a *n'anga*) argue as to whether it was the children of a witch or the witch herself who was sent out at night to lick people's plates so that, when they ate off them in the morning, they would be bewitched.

I am not given to fears of the supernatural but I recall being quite startled one night. It was 3.00 A.M. on a Sunday morning and I was attending a *bira* at which four *n'anga* were trying to make the spirit troubling a patient speak out. I was pretty tired and the *mbira* and drums, the beer and the dancing, had taken their toll. I sat in the round house (the healer's "clinic") near the door, quietly dozing. Suddenly the music became frantic, the *n'anga* coughed like a lion, the women ululated, and the chief *n'anga,* clad in the paraphenalia of his profession, leapt across the room toward me in an apparently impossible fashion. He had been sitting on the ground with his legs stretched out before him and now he was leaping across the floor in the same posture with his elbows flapping like a chicken's wings. I nearly drew on the "pooled imaginings" of those present to impute strange powers to him. There was a moment. . . .

The *n'anga* offer no story of the origin of evil: they simply say, "We are born into knowing it." Jealousy and envy are seen to be the most powerful motivating forces of evil. However, evil is also said to exist "for the sake of it." One's shades protect one against evil but, where the armor has chinks, evil slips in. We have seen that the effects of evil can be experienced by any member of the wider kin group if either a dead or a living kinsman has a grudge, or a debt, or has behaved immorally at any time. Difficult to keep the armor well oiled.

Before classifying the major guises that evil can take in Zezuru cosmology, I shall draw from anthropologists' generalizations on witchcraft and sorcery in Africa. Fortes describes them thus:

> The alleged witch is unaware of his or her evil propensities until accused and convicted. A witch then confesses to all the unnatural, immoral, sacrilegious and perverse habits that negate ordinary humanity, and characterize witchcraft—killing a child or a sibling for a feast of the witches' coven, flying by night to consume the soul or the womb or the potency of victims, committing incest, consorting with animal and other evil familiars, and so on. Such fantasies of sexual aggression and perversion, of soul cannibalism and of gross immorality that signifies their repudiation of normal humanity, are common in African witchcraft beliefs. [1987, 213]

Evans-Pritchard (1937) was the first anthropologist to clearly distinguish between witchcraft and sorcery in Africa: a witch is said to possess an inherited power that is used only for evil ends, whereas a sorcerer has the power to manipulate and alter natural and supernatural events with the proper magical knowledge and performance of ritual. Marwick defines other differences between witches and sorcerers:

As to motive, witches are considered to be slaves of aberration and addiction, and, thus conceived, are weird, sometimes tragic, figures. Sorcerers, on the other hand, are considered to be ordinary people driven to understandable, even if disapproved, urges, such as malice, envy or revenge, which are part of everyone's experience. [1982, 12–13]

In general, these descriptions hold for Zezuru notions of witchcraft and sorcery, although the defining lines are not always easy to trace. A witch may act consciously or unconsciously, but she (most are said to be female) does not only act at night. Probably she draws on mystical powers, but she can learn through apprenticeship to a practicing witch. Witches use medicine to make themselves invisible, to open the doors of other people's homes at night, to keep people asleep, and to smear on them or force them to drink while asleep. Chavunduka has done some fascinating work (unpublished) with confessed witches that confirms the above observations. Chavunduka (1982, 5) gives a broad definition for the Zezuru word for a witch—*muroyi* (plural, *varoyi*). It means a witch, a sorcerer, a poisoner, a person who fails to carry out the necessary rituals for his dead relatives, a person who commits an antisocial act, or even just a troublemaker. He notes that when pressed to distinguish between a witch and a sorcerer, the Zezuru usually describe a witch as one who operates at night and a sorcerer as one who operates during the day (23). Chavunduka (10) counts three types of witches: one who is possessed by an ancestral spirit who was a witch; another who is possessed by an alien spirit; and one who is sponsored by a practicing witch. Bourdillon notes that "normally it is assumed that the witches who teach the new witch her craft also provide her with a helping spirit" (1987b, 178).

Zezuru anticipate that misfortune may strike from the dead (via the ancestral spirits, alien spirits, or aggrieved spirits) or the living (witches or sorcerers) or natural causes. My concern in this chapter is not directly with the ancestral spirits—except those of former witches—because they are not seen to be evil. Fortes (1987) suggests that ancestors "are essentially projections of the jural authority vested in parents" (193) and are "comparable to externalized representations of conscience" (197) or "metaphorically speaking, an externalized superego" (211).

Evil is associated with witchcraft—"the paradigm of all evil and anti-social behaviour" (Bourdillon 1987b, 183)—and is performed by witches or sorcerers who may or may not have helping spirits. These spirits may be *midzimu* (ancestral) or *mashave* (alien) or *ngozi* (aggrieved). Bourdillon (ibid., 235) says that, theoretically the action of an angry spirit (*ngozi*) is quite distinct from witchcraft in that the former is usually thought to be the righteous action of an offended spirit—a physical evil, rather than the moral evil that witchcraft is. However, he adds, "Of all evil influences, an angry spirit (*ngozi*) is perhaps the most greatly feared by Shona" (235). For this reason and because a *ngozi* may be some alien spirit aroused by a witch, I treat their effects as falling within the range of evil forces.

Given the power and variety of sources of evil, it is not surprising that one healer could say, "The child is in the vortex of a battle between good and evil spirits as they compete for influence over the living." It is commonly said, and these beliefs are not kept secret from children, that witches are very fond of eating human flesh, especially the flesh of children; that in propitiating their spirits witches perform evil rites that may include the sacrifice of a baby; that the children of witches are all suspect; that a witch kills her own first born; and that witches cause newborn children to appear dead, then steal them from their graves and turn them into familiars. Some people say that witches' spirits tend to possess girls but kill off boys. Sleepwalking in children or mental retardation may be interpreted as signs of witchcraft affecting a child. The cause must be divined by a *n'anga*. Thus a child is likely to be made aware that supernatural evil exists and that it can affect the living. No child alone can ward off evil: protection depends on kin and community.

In the old days, people say, if a child fell seriously ill and witchcraft was suspected, the case became the concern of everyone in the village. Every woman had to cook porridge and feed a spoonful to the child, the assumption being that the witch would add an antidote to her porridge to avoid being exposed. If the child recovered, no further steps would be taken. Sometimes ordeals were held. In one such, the suspect was made to drink poison that caused the mouth and throat to swell; she was only given an antidote on confessing her sins. *N'anga* are said to hammer nails into the heads of witches caught doing nefarious deeds. Some families only discover that a kinswoman was a witch on her death, when a nail is seen in her head at the funeral.

In the following situation a *n'anga,* Chihata, tells a child's mother how to hammer a nail into a witch's head. I shall give a fair slice of the transcript because it illustrates how a child's condition is related to the family situation and to his or her talents. The case was openly examined in front of the patient, a ten-year-old boy, and children from the healer's homestead.

The boy was brought by his mother to Chihata because he was suffering from dizziness and stomach pains. When he was six weeks old his mother had found incisions on his navel. A *n'anga* had divined witchcraft but assured the boy's mother that if she applied the medicine he prescribed to protect his fontanelle he would come to no harm. When the boy was two years of age, another attempt to bewitch him was made and the same *n'anga* cleansed him. The boy was well until he turned seven, when he became dizzy, had weak legs, and would lose consciousness for short periods. He had suffered thus for three years. Here is a transcript from the consultation.

Chihata uses a glass jar, into which she peers and sees "visions." She looks into her jar and asks the boy's mother: "Do cats come around the homestead at night?"

Mother agrees.

Chihata: "They cry [imitates the cry] like a baby?"

Mother agrees:

Chihata: "The boy is bright—there may be jealousy. There is a snake that comes to your home and wants to sleep in your blankets. Did you see it?"

Mother: "Yes. A girl in our homestead saw it as it was entering and my husband killed it."

Chihata: "You have fooled yourselves: it is still alive."

Mother: "There are no cracks for a snake to enter our bedroom."

Chihata: "You are cheating yourself. There are no barriers to witchcraft. A snake can even emerge through the floor. The snake was sent to place things in the boy's body. The witch uses the snake as a belt."

Mother: "I have consulted different *n'anga* and they all agree."

Chihata [consults her glass]: "I have also seen that this woman is a showoff and arouses jealousy." [Mother laughs.]

Mother: "I have worked hard. I have earned enough for a sewing machine."

Chihata: "Even to sew a single stitch you charge ten cents! Your only solution is to remove the child from this area."

[A long discussion of the boy's health, education, and hospital treatment and of the possibility of his living in Harare follows.]

Mother: "If the boy must go to Harare, I will not disrupt his education now but will send him next year."

Chihata: "You will carry his bones to Harare."

Mother: "If he goes, I will have no one to help with the cattle. There is no one to care for him there except his father."

[The *n'anga* shrugs and gives the boy's mother advice on how to overcome a witch. She draws a line at the base and the top of her door.]

Chihata: "Do that and say out, 'Anyone who saw his or her father's or mother's childhood come and stand at the door.' This prevents the witch from coming through. Scatter the herb that causes dizziness. Don't be afraid as you do it. If you scream or cry out, you will die."

Mother: "I will be afraid."

Chihata: "As you do it, a vision of the witch will come to you. If a person comes to the door, he or she will be glued to the medicine. Hold him and hammer a nail into the head. The vision is the person. He will then make the coughing sound of one possessed and walk away. A witch does not die. The person will be ill and when he dies people will see on the head a nail or a hole which will identify him as a witch. He will not live long as a bone is cracked in the head."

[The children's eyes were, by this time, as large as owls'.]

Another *n'anga* described a patient's story that reflects on a child's duty to his or her parent(s) even in the face of suspicions of witchcraft:

A woman was living with her son and his wife. The son suspected that his mother was "coming between me and my wife at night." He consulted a *n'anga,* who gave him medicine "to see at night." The next night he "saw" his mother sleeping naked beside him. When he asked her what she was doing in his room, she stood up and went to her own. The man's wife fell ill and was hospitalized. While on the operating table, evil medicine came out of her nose and she died.

A *gata* (a ritual to divine the cause of death) was held and kin from both families attended. The chief *n'anga* called up the spirit of the dead woman and she challenged the mother-in-law. It emerged that the latter was jealous of her daughter-in-law's sway over her son and suspected that she was turning him against her. She and another daughter-in-law poisoned her at night, feeding her evil medicine through her mouth while she slept.

Like the spirits, parents must be treated with care and respect, but they can cause great harm when motivated by emotions like jealousy. Of course, no parent would harm a child unless she or he had already dabbled in evil. In the above story, the son knew of his mother's witchcraft but could not turn against a parent. As the *n'anga* explained, "It is impossible to reject one's parents." Once the evil becomes public, the matter is taken out of the hands of those directly involved. In times gone by, the community would, the *n'anga* said, have put the woman suspected of witchcraft through an ordeal. If a child turns against a parent, the parent, after death, will return to trouble him or her as a *ngozi*: if the community or senior kinsmen handle the case, this will not happen (see appendix 12, on witchcraft accusations that came to my attention in 1982 in Musami).

The reverse holds true: if a parent turns on a child, he or she must expect retaliation from the ancestors. Even if a woman aborts a fetus, she could be troubled by *ngozi*. A parent does not have unlimited powers over a child for, Zezuru say, "Children belong to the spirits." Western medical personnel often cause distress when they accuse parents of bringing sick children for treatment too long after symptoms have appeared; they set aside with scorn the parents' pleas that the ancestors had to be consulted first.

To conclude the last two sections on identity and evil, I suggest that a Zezuru child is introduced to shared notions of supernatural evil that *can* conjure up an atmosphere to terrify him or her. However, when the child has a healthy family and community structure and a firm sense of identity, the terror is seldom actualized. When things go awry an idiom of malevolence exists that can be used to bracket distress. Fortes says that while the Tallensi recognize the existence of evil, they "relegate the notion of witchcraft to a marginal and relatively dormant symbolical role in their theory of human nature and of causality" (1987, 212). He attributes their "denial of magical power to destructive human impulses to the integrity of individual identity owing to the incorporation by the individual of the family structure" (ibid.). In contrast, the Ashanti believe that witchcraft operates "in the framework of close matrilineal kinship like a self-destructive, self-hating power" (214). Fortes refers the Ashanti readiness to accept and use witchcraft beliefs "to their insecure sense of identity due to the conflicting patterns of authority, responsibility and nurturance with which the individual grows up" (215). The idiom in which evil is expressed is, in the opinion of Fortes, shaped by identity. Ngubane (1977, 147–49) takes the expression of individual deviance as evidenced in evil possession and relates it to social malady:

> What I am suggesting here is that the notion of evil spirit possession is used among the Zulu as an idiom to handle the escalating proportions of psychoneurosis often associated with failure to cope with the changing way of life in the colonial and post-colonial industrial society. [149]

How the expression of evil is interpreted has grave implications for the process of healing. Ideas of guilt, sin, personal culpability, identity, dependence, and destiny are acquired by children and internalized. Therapy that fails to place illness within the context of cosmology loses efficacy. A person is a tree that can be shaken at any time.

CONCLUSION

The Turn of the Screw ends with a scene between the governess and Miles. She confronts him with her understanding of the evil forces that have him under their power. She again "sees" the apparitions and attempts to "shield" the boy. The scene builds to a climax of horror and ends with these final words from the manuscript, said to have been written by the governess: "We were alone with the quiet day, and his little heart, dispossessed, had stopped" (550).

Yet again James taunts the reader with ambiguity. Was the boy a victim of his governess's malevolent imaginings? Was he a sacrifice? Did he even see the apparitions? Was he dispossessed? We are left with only the fact of his death on a quiet day. We have seen that in Zezuru terms, the governess set about expelling the evil in a ham-handed fashion. Bourdillon notes that, among the Shona, once an angry spirit has become active, it must be appeased, and "the mediumship of a diviner specialized in dealing with avenging spirits is usually required (an unspecialized diviner would not dare to meddle in the affairs of an angry spirit for fear of bringing its anger upon himself)" (1987b, 234). The governess dared to meddle and the boy died.

Underlying Zezuru concepts of evil are the following axioms. That the transition from childhood to adulthood is the transition from innocence to a social identity and integrity of self. Evildoers are adults who have failed to achieve that transition according to the norms and ethics of their community. The victims of evil are often the innocent (children) and inadequate (adults). Healing aims to establish, reestablish, and strengthen a workable social identity and integrity of self. Evil (as expressed in witchcraft, possession, etc.) is part of a discourse on human suffering—illness, misfortune, death—operative within a specific community. And, finally, the integrity of that community is critical for its well-being and that of its constituent individuals: without integrity the community's ethical code cracks and its discourse falls apart.

Traditional healers in Mashonaland take notions of evil into account in their diagnosis and treatment of patients. Community is the crucial context for the efficacy of therapy: yet we must pay attention in order to hear the child's message. If we do not understand the nuances that surround any episode of illness, we will be unable to penetrate defenses, or receive hidden messages, or listen with understanding to a sick or troubled child.

CHAPTER FIVE

CHILDREN ON HERBS,
HEALING, AND HEALERS

IF, AS the chapters in this volume suggest, learning to heal often begins in childhood, and if some children are given the opportunity to learn about herbs and healing from healers within the family, and if healers reflect in their practices the conceptions of childhood current among their clients, then a series of questions relating to children's experiences and thinking present themselves. Are there differences among children in their knowledge of and concern with healing? Do those who live with healers have a greater practical knowledge of herbs? Do children articulate their communities' formulations about religion that underscore the healing enterprise? This chapter complements the concerns of those that precede it. To understand the theories, knowledge, ethical ideas, and practices of *n'anga* it may be fruitful to examine children's theories and knowledge.

Children reflect on social norms. Their reflections may underscore lines of stress and changing mores. They may also show how the nuances of symbolic expression are transmitted across generations. By investigating children's knowledge of plants used for medicinal and ritual purposes (for brevity's sake I shall refer to all the plants as herbs), I hoped to describe children's practical interests in the business of healing. And by interviewing children, I hoped to elicit their ideas about healing. Some children are provided with the opportunity and encouragement to acquire specialized skills and information to do with healing. The first section examines these possibilities. It begins with a summary of some of the ideas presented earlier in this book.

WHAT N'ANGA LOOK FOR

When *n'anga* look for children to assist them, they select children with good hearts (which includes estimates of their trustworthiness, moral fiber, and their ability to behave quietly and sensibly). After that, they select those who show interest. Interest, they say, is the prime ingredient for success in learning to heal. Chihata said, "One is always clever in what one is interested in."[1]

Mande, in explaining why his one son can invoke Mande's spirit while his other sons cannot, said that the ability is to do with the individual's interest. Compatibility is another criteria of selection: there should be sufficient liking for a bond to develop (the word used to describe such mutual understanding is *kuwirirana*—to be at one, in agreement, mutually well disposed).

However, most *n'anga* adamantly claim that it is useless to teach a child unless he or she has already been selected by a spirit, often at this stage by a *mashave*. Healers say they cannot ensure the passing on of their stock of knowledge because it is the spirits who control both the selection and training of persons in each generation. They also say that if a child expresses interest it implies the presence of a *shave*. The theory circles in upon itself. Healers select children they think are bright and able and with whom they have mutual understanding. Children may show interest, thus suggesting that spiritual attention has focused on them.

As it is widely said that healers are not trained and that healing spirits pass over one generation between those whom they possess, I was surprised to find how many healers teach their own children. The fourteen healers in Musami whose families I know particularly well had trained nineteen of their children to act as acolytes. Of the nine-

---

[1]Karl Popper thinks similarly: he says that what characterizes creative thinking is "the intensity of the interest in the problem" (1976, 40).

teen, twelve were sons and seven daughters. Seven of the males were
adult in 1982–1983, as were five of the females. The same healers also
depended on one husband, two wives, one mother, one sister's son,
and nine grandchildren (three boys and six girls) to assist them. That
is, thirty-three family members had, at one time or another, been
drawn into the healing enterprise. None of the healers expected their
own children to be possessed by their healing spirits after their death
but some thought that the grandchildren might inherit their spirits.
Their own children could, of course, inherit spirits from their ancestors or be possessed by *mashave* (including *njuzu*) or even *mhondoro*
or *gombwe* spirits.

CHILDREN AS ASSISTANTS

The Zezuru word for an acolyte is *nechombo,* which can mean senior grandson or interpreter of a medium (Hannan 1984, 445). (The
word *makumbi*—a female diviner-healer, or wife of a diviner-healer,
or assistant—is used by Gelfand et al. 1985.) I use *nechombo* here to
mean attendant, assistant, or novice. Healers seldom work all alone.
One reason is that when a healer is possessed the spirit takes over and
the healer is said to be unaware of what he or she is saying or doing.
Very often the spirit's actions and words have to be translated for the
patient(s) by an acolyte. The acolyte also informs the healer when he
or she comes out of the trance. The presence of an acolyte adds to the
air of importance and mystery. Some healers treat only with a third
party present, to prevent the possibility of a patient's accusations of
abuse, especially sexual. Also, healers with busy practices need help in
collecting herbs and preparing medicines. Acolytes are sometimes
sent alone into the bush to gather herbs. They may treat patients according to healers' instructions while the healers are away. Patients
usually present themselves first to an acolyte, who then conducts
them into the healer's presence.

While many of these tasks are menial, the acolytes watch and
listen. They participate in consultations and rituals that encompass a
broad range of the people's concerns. During a healer's career, more
adults and children participate in the healing process than the norms

about learning would indicate. At any one point, a fair number of people with some experience in working with healers can be called upon to come forward to direct ritual procedures.

The following description of the selection of a child to act as acolyte for a healer in Musami is given to illustrate the care that often goes into the selection.

Makumbi is possessed by her father's mother's spirit. She specializes in treating stomach troubles, problems that relate to babies' vulnerabilities to illness, and the effects of evil forces diagnosed in the condition of the fontanelle, and infertility. She grew up with her grandmother, who was a healer. Beside the spirit of an ancestor, she is possessed by two *mashave.* Makumbi trained her eldest daughter as her acolyte. The daughter, aged eighteen in 1982, subsequently trained as a Red Cross assistant. Two of Makumbi's younger children, a boy of fourteen and a girl of twelve, help her sometimes.

The process whereby an acolyte is chosen in this family is unusual. Makumbi's husband's kin select a child to work closely with her. "This," she says, "is to avoid problems resulting from mishandling herbs." When her eldest daughter left home, Makumbi's in-laws conducted a ritual to break her ties to her mother. Another small ritual will be held to initiate a new helper. A pot of beer will be passed to Makumbi, and in accepting it she signifies her acceptance of their selection. The compliance of the child is not sought. The selection is based on the child's behavior: qualities such as quietness, decency, and obedience are sought.

Her fourteen-year-old son may have a spirit seeking to possess him. He cried and walked so late (he was two years old before he could walk) that a diviner was consulted. It was divined that the boy's father's father wanted the boy to be named after him. A ritual with beer was held and black beads were tied around the small child's wrists. He soon cried less and began to walk. His mother says that he now loves to be with a group of dogs and may have a hunting *shave.*

The involvement of Makumbi's husband's kin in her healing profession is more direct than is usually the case. However, in-laws often demand most of the earnings from a daughter-in-law who treats patients. Perhaps Makumbi's spirit was taking revenge when she was unable to breastfeed her last child. During a *bira* her in-laws were blamed for not having thanked the spirit for the safe delivery of the child at home.

A TEST OF CHILDREN'S KNOWLEDGE OF PLANTS

To determine whether children who live with a healer learn more about plants used for medicinal and ritual purposes than do children who do not live with a healer, I devised a test to administer to two groups. Forty-eight children were tested. Twenty-four children (twelve girls and twelve boys) made up the sample and they were drawn from among those who live with a healer.[2] They ranged in age from six to seventeen and were in Grades One to Form One at the local schools. They were matched in terms of sex, age, and grade with children drawn from one of the local schools, Mabika School.[3] This second group, also composed of twelve girls and twelve boys, made up the control group. There were no distinguishing characteristics between the sample and the control groups except that the former lived with at least one *n'anga* who was a close relative and the latter did not.

The forty-eight children grew up in the countryside, but Musami is not far from the country's capital city, Harare. Most of their fathers worked in the city, but many returned to Musami at the weekends. Their fathers worked as policemen, clerks, firemen, drivers, mechanics, tailors, builders, cashiers, waiters, and in other similar jobs. These occupations suggest secure positions within the lower middle class

---

[2]In Reynolds (1986, 176) there is a reference to twenty-five children in each group. In later analysis I canceled one from each, as two children were too young (five years old).

[3]I am grateful to the headmaster, Mr. P. C. T. Chingwaro, and his staff for allowing me to administer the tests at Mabika School, and to R. B. Drummond and S. Mave of the National Botanical Gardens for helping me identify the scientific names of the plants.

and better salaries than many rural families would have achieved under the Rhodesian regime. One-fifth of the children's fathers were farmers. The children's own ambitions expressed hopes for achievement beyond their fathers'. Nineteen wanted to become teachers, nine nurses, seven doctors, four car mechanics, and two engineers. The rest wanted to be clerks, train drivers, nuns, pilots, bookkeepers, *n'anga,* and so on. The children described their mothers as housewives or farmers (or both). Few of their mothers worked in the city.

Most of the children came from large families. Again the sample group did not differ from the control group. Eighty percent came from families of five to ten children and 20 percent from families of one to four children. Or, to phrase this differently, 15 percent had seven to nine siblings, 66 percent had four to six, and 20 percent had one to three. There was a fairly even spread of children in terms of their birth order, although only one was the eighth born and two the ninth born in their families.

Only eleven of the children said that they lived with both parents (because their fathers lived in the city). Twenty-five lived with their mothers and eleven with their grandparents (this usually included the mother too, and the grandparents were most often the father's parents). The fathers of four children had died. One child lived with her mother's elder sister.

In summary, the children in the sample and in the control groups shared similar backgrounds. They lived among kin in a relatively prosperous area from which the men traveled to work, living away from home but returning often. Each family had access to land on which both cash and subsistence crops were grown.

Of the twenty-four children in the sample, fifteen lived with a mother who was a healer, one with a father, one with a father's brother, eight with a mother's mother, two with a father's father, and one with a mother's father. That is, the children lived with twenty-eight healers, of whom seventeen were of the parental generation and eleven of the grandparental generation; four children lived with members of both generations who heal.

The test consisted of two parts. In the first part (Test A) each child was presented, in private, with pieces of root, bark, stem, and leaf of eleven plants. These were laid out on a table. The child was asked to name the plants, say what each was used for, identify the part used, and describe the preparation and administration of the medicine. A point was earned for each step correctly given. The total possible score was 44. The eleven plants were chosen by four healers as being in use for medicinal purposes in the area. Each healer confirmed the identity and use of the selected plants. The Shona names by which the plants are known in the Musami area are *mudima, murungu, mupfeyo, musvisvinwa, mukuvazviyo, musikavakadzi, muroro, muwore, zheverashuro, mufufu,* and *bepu.* The four healers in Musami gave a range of uses for the selected plants, all of which fall within those identified for use by Gelfand et al. (1985). Appendix 13 gives the plants' scientific names, and references to Wild (1972) and Gelfand et al. (1985) where descriptions, uses, and preparations of the plants by Shona healers can be found.

Test A was difficult. Whole plants were not given; the children had to identify them by pieces of bark, stem, or root, or by a leaf (many of the leaves of the plants are similar). Cunningham observes that in Natal few urban traders and herbalists are prosecuted for "selling 'specially protected species' as few white conservation officers can classify any of the bewildering array of dried bark, roots or bulbs according to species" (1988, 25).

In the second part of the test (Test B), each child was given a basket and requested to collect plants from the bush that he or she recognized as being used for medicine. The child was awarded points for bringing any plant that matched our sample and identifying it as such, for naming a plant, giving its use, identifying the part used, and describing the preparation and administration. The four *n'anga* checked the children's collections for me.

Tables 1 and 2 give the results. Points earned by boys and girls were remarkably similar. Children who live with healers scored more on Test A and Test B and overall. The children named 68 plants as having uses that they identified. Some of the children could have collected many more plants about whose use they know had we allowed sufficient time. That is to say, the real depth of their pharmacopoeia was not plumbed. The level of difficulty in Test A was very high and scores were low; however, one girl and one boy in the sample scored 31.8 per cent and 43.2 percent of the total possible score.

While the results confirm my hypothesis that children living with

RESULTS

Table 1: Test of Plants and their Uses Administered to Two Groups of Children

Sample: Children who live with healers						Control: Children who do not live with healers			
Girls:				Test Results				Test Results	
No.	Age	Grade	A	B	Total	No.	A	B	Total
1	6	1	2	1	3	25	0	0	0
2	7	1	0	0	0	26	0	0	0
3	7	1	0	2	2	27	6	12	18
4	7	1	0	3	3	28	0	0	0
5	9	2	6	6	12	29	0	2	2
6	11	3	4	8	12	30	8	8	16
7	11	4	0	10	10	31**	7	21	28
8*	12	5	6	27	33	32	0	3	3
9	12	5	4	22	26	33	1	7	8
10	13	6	5	8	13	34	8	16	24
11*	16	6	9	25	34	35	4	15	19
12	14	6	14	29	43	36	0	7	7
			50	141	191		34	91	125
Boys									
13	7	1	0	3	3	37	0	0	0
14	8	2	0	10	10	38+	4	8	12
15	10	2	4	8	12	39	4	8	12
16	8	3	7	2	9	40	0	8	8
17	12	4	0	8	8	41	0	12	12
18	13	5	0	20	20	42	4	4	8
19*	13	7	4	23	27	43	4	8	12
20	14	Form 1	5	8	13	44	3	12	15
21*	14	Form 1	19	33	52	45	1	11	12
22	16	Form 1	1	14	15	46	0	12	12
23	16	Form 1	0	14	14	47	8	12	20
24	16	Form 1	0	13	13	48	9	12	21
			40	156	196		37	107	144

*These children acted as acolytes to healers in their families.
**This child has a *svikiro* (diviner) in the family though not living with her.
+ This child's mother's sister is a *n'anga* but does not live with them.

Table 2: Summary of Scores and Percentages

	Test A		Test B		Tests A & B	
	Scores	Percent of Total Score	Scores	Percent of Total Score	Scores	Percent of Total Score
Sample	90	56	294	60	384	59
Control	71	44	198	40	269	41
Total	161	100	492	100	653	100

healers learn more about plants for medicinal purposes, I was surprised at the range of knowledge displayed by many of the children in both groups. I suggest that this finding supports another hypothesis, namely that knowledge of healing and ritual that includes a broad-based knowledge of plants and their uses is widespread. Diviners and healers operate within communities of people well versed in ritual procedure and plant lore. I did not anticipate that this spread of knowledge would be revealed by tests conducted among children. The implications of this claim are far-reaching. If *n'anga* do not hold a monopoly on knowledge (especially of materia medica) and if people monitor their performance, diagnosis, and treatment from a basis of understanding, then it is false to separate the experience and practice of *n'anga* too clearly from that of the population.

CHILDREN'S CONCEPTIONS OF HEALING

Thirty-six children who live in the Musami area were interviewed on their conceptions of healing, the roles of *n'anga,* and related cosmological issues. Fifteen were the children or grandchildren of healers and lived with a healer: the other twenty-one had no healer living in their homesteads and no close kin who practiced healing. Seven of the former group and eight of the latter had participated in the herb test. There were more older children among those interviewed than those tested. They ranged in age from seven to seventeen and they were in classes from Grade Two to Form Three, all at local schools. Half of them were in primary and half in secondary school.

The interview covered six topics: personal experiences of *n'anga;* how a person becomes a *n'anga;* conceptions of evil; conceptions of witchcraft and sorcery; of traditional and western healing; and on their experiences during the war. There were sixty-five questions. Each child was interviewed alone and in chiShona. The children participated cheerfully and seemed to be keen to express their ideas.

The children were more articulate about these issues than I had anticipated. They had a much wider range of understanding of and involvement in conceptions to do with healing, training, the origin of evil, the source of witchcraft, and similar matters than I had expected. A few of the older children attempted to adopt a "modern" stance expressing scorn for and disinterest in "traditional" ideas. However, they were unable to sustain that position. They soon became deeply immersed in explaining cosmological concerns of Zezuru people derived from ideas formulated long ago. I shall briefly describe the replies (their experiences during the war are reported on elsewhere in this volume).

Personal Experiences of N'anga

Most of the children said that they personally know *n'anga* (78 percent) and nearly half of them named one or more healers. Only a quarter (26 percent) admitted to having visited a healer for treatment or advice, and another 9 percent said that family members had consulted healers on their behalf. Over four questions it turned out that some 40 percent of the children had visited a *n'anga* either for their own consultation or a family member's consultation or had had a family member consult a healer on their behalf. That is, nearly half the children had experience of a healer's advice.

No child said that he or she had had a dream interpreted by a healer (one boy dreamed of his aunt and shoe polish, and his brother interpreted the dream as predicting a new pair of shoes, but their mother, a *n'anga,* laughed at the dream and the interpretation). However, a third of the children remembered dreams that had been interpreted by their elders. One child's dream of brightly colored fish was said to foretell a windfall of money, as was another's. A girl dreamed that she died and this was taken as a warning of death in the family and, not long thereafter, her sister's son died; another child dreamed of the death of an uncle (*baba makura*), but no clear interpretation was given; yet another dreamed of building and the dream was said to foretell a death—and, indeed, the child's aunt (*amanini*) died. Yet another girl dreamed of a snake on her back but was not told the interpretation given by her grandmother.

The children of healers related five dreams that had been interpreted by their elders. Their dreams resonated with the symbols seen by *n'anga* to presage the presence of spirits. One was of repeated drownings and rescues by birds; another set were of swimming; a third was of hunting; a fourth of plowing (this was said to predict a death in the family, but the child says that nobody died); and the fifth was of jumping from a mountain and landing safely. The last set of dreams was said to predict spiritual possession of the child in the near future—he was at the time aged seventeen and his mother, mother's mother, and father's brother were *n'anga*.

Almost all the children (89 percent) had attended at least one ritual at which one or more *n'anga* presided. Marked differences in the experience of children in the two groups (those with healers in their immediate families and those without) showed up in their replies to questions on collecting herbs with *n'anga*, preparing medicines, helping to treat patients, and acting as acolytes. Of the former group, 67 percent said that they had been involved in one or more of these tasks, while none of the latter group said that he or she had.

How a Person Becomes a N'anga

No child believed that someone can simply decide to become a *n'anga*. Most of the children said that a person must be possessed by an ancestral or *njuzu* spirit and taught about healing through dreams. Two suggested that the ability is inherited, four that it can be learned from *n'anga*, and three that it can be bought, although each child suggested this rather tentatively and in relation to an alternative—that is, possession or learning from healers. Thirteen children, including the four mentioned above, said that a person can be taught to heal if he or she shows signs of being possessed, especially via dreams. Children, then, express the same range of options as do adults: none feel that one can simply elect to become a *n'anga;* almost all say that spiritual possession is a prerequisite; many mention dreams as the main conduit; and a surprisingly large number said that one can be taught to heal—surprising because this is not the received wisdom. In describing the process through which people pass in order to become healers the children of *n'anga* mentioned sickness more often than did the other children. Again, the range was wide and the process was said to include dreams, experience, tutelage, and training by *njuzu* while under the water. One child suggested that in order to survive the process one needed to be very stubborn.

The children said that Shona people have different kinds of healers, and they named those possessed by *vadzimu, njuzu,* and *mashave,* and those who use *hakaka.* Children of *n'anga* mentioned a wider variety of techniques that distinguish healers—sucking out evil, knowledge of herb properties, dreams, using a mirror, and experience in healing.

Two questions asked whether there are differences between *n'anga* and *chiremba* and between *chiremba* and *svikiro* (the words most often used in reference to traditional healers in the area; see Appendix 14 for a discussion of the terms used in the literature). The children were asked to describe the differences, if there were any. The children's explanations reflect the confusion that exists among adults (including academics). Just over half the children said that *n'anga* and *chiremba* are the same. The others gave a variety of reasons as to why they are different: a quarter said a *chiremba* is a Western doctor; some that only *n'anga* divine; and some that only *chiremba* divine. Almost all the children said the terms *chiremba* and *svikiro* have different meanings. Many said that *chiremba* heal without being possessed and *svikiro* divine through possession. Some thought that *svikiro* are only prophets and advisors; others, that they learn about herbs from spirits and heal, while *chiremba* are instructed by other healers on plant lore, then heal. Over half the children of healers said that *svikiro* are possessed but do not heal. Some said *chiremba* are possessed and that they heal but do not divine.

On whether or not children can be possessed by healing spirits and whether or not signs are given to children presaging future possession, all but one of the children of healers said they could be possessed and are given signs. In the other group, just over half said the same. The signs include illness, odd behavior, knowledge of herbs while still a child, behavior as if possessed, nightmares, fears, bravery, dreams from the spirits, naughtiness, and the rejection of particular foods or other things like the use of petroleum jelly or perfume. Nineteen of all the children described a child known to them who is either possessed or who shows powerful signs of future possession (eleven of these were the children of *n'anga*). The children said to be possessed or identified for future possession were aged ten to seventeen, and eleven of them were boys. Only two of the children interviewed said that they did not know about these matters, and only six firmly said that children could not be possessed nor show signs of future possession.

Children laid heavy emphasis on the importance of dreams as

means for instructing healers about the healing properties of plants—over half of them say healers learn about herbs through dreams. Nearly half say healers are instructed by spirits; a quarter by other healers; and a few mention other forces including God, snuff, and ritual occasions. Half the children of *n'anga* were very sure that learning comes from both the spirit world and other *n'anga*.

On Evil

The answers to this set of questions were well articulated, and there seemed to be little difference between the conceptions held by children who live with healers and those who do not. On the origin of evil in a person, the children blamed inheritance (43 percent); *ngozi* (40 percent); nature or Satan (9 percent); witches (6 percent); poverty (6 percent); one blamed parents for failing to teach their children well; and some did not know (17 percent). The next question asked, "If a person does something very bad—like killing someone—but is not found out, will that person still be punished in some way?" I was inquiring about notions of retribution from the spirit world. A quarter of the respondents thought that no punishment would follow (only one child of a healer thought thus). Two-thirds believed that retribution would follow through *ngozi*, and a tenth through God or an ancestor, who would inform the police, or revelation in dreams or divination by a *n'anga*.

On being asked "What is *ngozi?*" every child gave a clear reply. Their definitions included the following:

The spirit of a person who died with a grudge and comes back to seek revenge.

An evil spirit that was wronged while alive and returns to seek payment.

The spirit of a murdered person which comes back to torment the murderer.

One who comes back to torment his murderer or his family. Makes them a bit mentally unfit.

Ngozi is when one beats or insults one's mother. Mother dies
and comes back to torment you.

Like me, I would come back to you and you would be seeing my
vision everywhere you look.

On Witchcraft and Sorcery

The children suggested a number of ways that a person can become
a witch. Half the children believed that witches are possessed by ancestral or alien spirits (50 percent); a quarter of them thought that the
evil powers could be bought (25 percent); some thought a witch could
learn through apprenticeship (14 percent); and a few that a witch is
created by Satan or uses knowledge about herbs for evil ends.

In replying to questions on whether or not they had had witches
pointed out to them or been affected by witchcraft or seen its effect
on kin or neighbors, over half the children replied that they had not
(58 percent). Of those, 47 percent lived with healers and 58 percent did
not. However, every child answered subsequent questions in a way
that affirmed his or her fear of witches. The children cited twenty
cases in which witchcraft was said to have caused illness or misfortune to the child him or herself or kin or neighbors. One of the group
of children who do not live with healers told us of two cases. In one, a
woman who suffered constant headaches was diagnosed as having
been bewitched. A *n'anga* sucked out a metal nut and pieces of a tire
from her head. In the other case, the respondent's elder sister was
bewitched—she cried with body and head pains. Her mother took her
to a *n'anga,* who sucked out a baby's finger and a needle from her
body. The witch's complexion and the position of her homestead
were described. She was no relation.

Over half the children said that one can protect oneself against
harm from witchcraft either by taking herbs or consulting a *n'anga.*
Only 22 percent felt there were no means to protect against witches'
harm. When asked directly if witchcraft is inherited no child replied
no. Ninety-two percent said it is. When asked if they would play with
the children of someone pointed out to be a witch, they gave a variety
of responses: some said no, they would be afraid; others yes, they
would fear annoying the family if they refused to play; and yet others

said that they would play with the children, as only one child is selected for training in witchcraft. Most children felt that they can do
nothing to frighten or chase a witch—some said witches are invisible
when operating—but 22 percent would make a direct attack if they
saw a witch in action. Over three-quarters of the children felt that
those who are particularly able in school or in sport are more vulnerable to the evil effects of witchcraft resulting from other people's
jealousy and should take precautions by protecting themselves. (Appendix 15 gives two reports from national newspapers on the scourge
of belief in witchcraft and on the effect of superstition on soccer
players.)

A third of the respondents felt that witchcraft would increase if
there were no *n'anga* to hold witches at bay. Finally, two-thirds of the
children said that *n'anga* can use their power or knowledge of medicines for evil ends (of those, half were children who live with *n'anga*).
During the interview four children expressed some skepticism about
the reality or force of traditional views of evil and mystical power.
None maintained this position for more than a few questions. The
children fear witchcraft and sorcery. They hold a similar range of views
about its source and expression as the adults in the community do.
The replies of children who lived with healers and those who did not
showed no marked differences. Among the latter, ten children mentioned thirteen cases of witchcraft.

Traditional and Western Healing

Eleven questions to do with the children's preferences and understanding of traditional and Western healing patterns were asked. I
shall give a summary of their responses. Seventy-one percent of the
sample group (children who live with *n'anga*) said that when they fall
ill they are first treated by Western healers (at hospitals or clinics)
and 95 percent of the control group said the same. Similarly, 7 percent
and 5 percent, respectively, were first taken to traditional healers.
Among the sample group, 21 percent said that they are as likely to be
treated first under either system. Given a choice, those who live with
n'anga gave more varied replies—29 percent would go to a Western
healer, 29 percent to a traditional healer, and 21 percent to either or
both. Their reasons included the following: Western healers give

"proper medication"; "I go to hospital as I am not happy about *n'anga*"; and "the clinic gives fast results." Traditional healers were preferred because "they give protective herbs and treat the illness so that it does not return"; because "I know what their medicines treat, whereas at the clinic they give useless injections—you might just die there"; because some *n'anga* "diagnose illness without being told by the patient what it is"; and because "I think they know more."

Children who do not live with healers were more certain in their choice of first consulting Western healers (71 percent), but most said that if they were not cured, they would consult *n'anga*. Only 14 percent said they would first visit a *n'anga*. Another 14 percent said they would consult a healer from either system for these reasons: "I don't mind: in the true sense they are all healers"; "They heal different illnesses"; and "I am not choosey. I would consult any that cure but I would always choose a *n'anga* even if I broke a limb, as a cure does not occur until witchcraft has been detected."

Both groups of children (86 percent and 71 percent, respectively) believe that there are problems that can only be handled by traditional healers (like witchcraft, fontanelle problems, spirit possession, *jeko*,[4] protection, and some women's illnesses). The children also believe (86 percent and 71 percent, respectively) that there are illnesses that can be cured only by Western healers (like schistosomiasis, fractures, eye, ear, and dental problems, cancer, tetanus, malaria, internal problems, problems needing operations or caused by accidents, and dizziness). Once again the children gave thoughtful replies.

CONCLUSION

I had anticipated greater differences between the two groups in their understanding of and attitudes toward the role traditional healers play in the cosmological whole. The main differences lay in the children's actual experience with the handling of materia medica or pa-

---

[4]*Jeko* is dysmenorrhea, or painful menstruation (Gelfand et al. 1985, 340).

tients. Both groups of children ranged in their views from credulity to skepticism. None consistently maintained a position of skepticism toward traditional beliefs in witchcraft, sorcery, or evil. Children in both groups demonstrated that they understood their society's formulations that involved good, evil, the relationships between a living person and a spirit, the manifestations of spirits among people, the means whereby knowledge and power are acquired, and the vulnerability of individuals.

A number of practical issues emerged from the interviews. One is that children feel vulnerable to personal attack by evil forces. Many feel that jealousy and envy give rise to attacks of witchcraft or sorcery: favored or talented children are particularly exposed. Children are also aware of the possibility that they are exposed to evil through the misdemeanors or crimes of adults. The newspaper article reprinted in appendix 16 is given to show that children's fears have a base, even if only in rare, aberrant behavior. This awareness must have implications for children's views of their own ability to protect themselves through moral purity. If they feel vulnerable to evil forces as expressed in physical or mental illness, then healers (especially those trained in the Western healing system) ought to be cognizant of the possible meanings that underlie symptom presentation. At the University of Zimbabwe a special committee has been formed to discuss whether or not students bringing certificates from traditional healers who have treated them for "*ngozi* problems" should be regarded as having been ill and therefore eligible for deferment of examinations, just as students bringing certificates from certified Western doctors or psychologists are. Is *ngozi* a "real" problem? If it is, can Western healers be expected to treat it seriously? If it is not "real," should students who claim to be troubled by *ngozi* be treated as mentally disturbed? And, if they are, who should certify them as such? It is a nice conundrum for academics to ponder.

I set out to discover what children know about herbs, healers, and healing and whether or not children related to healers know much more than others. And, in essence, I found that this kind of knowledge, which can be termed religious, is common sense—that is, known to a lot of children. But some are called and their learning goes beyond common sense into practice and the creation of their own special expertise and insight. A major point is that very few children "don't know" at the more general level.

A summary of the evidence and arguments presented in this chapter follows. First we looked at how children are selected as acolytes and saw that some are carefully chosen as assistants and some are seen to have been "called." The result is that particular relationships between *n'anga* and children result in the spread of a fairly wide range of expertise. A case study was given as illustration of this.

The next step was to examine how specialized this expertise is. This was done by means of a test among healer-related and non-healer-related children. The findings suggest that both groups are quite well informed on plants used for medicines. Nevertheless, the ultimate extent of the knowledge of some children who have worked with healers was not measured.

A third stage was to explore what expertise, apart from herbs, children have acquired. Here their concepts were researched. Important differences in the two groups were identified in their actual experience of handling medicines and treating patients. However, it was found that all the children share a general knowledge of the community's ideas about possession, vulnerability, inheritance, and other matters. In the range of their ideas and the individuality of their expression, it was clear that they were not repeating adult formulae, but had pondered carefully on many topics in relation to their own thoughts and experiences.

I suggest that this knowledge is available to children: available for all to delve into and for some to develop an interest in. The nature of the knowledge is common yet the practice is specialized. Children are aware that they can participate in this religious sphere, that there are a number of routes to extensive involvement, that actual practice is not the same as understanding, that understanding is necessary for their own safety, and that performance is risky. In part, I am suggesting that the young conceive of their distress and their need for security in religious terms. These terms frame their quest for relief. The quest can be seen in the context of the young people's sense of vulnerability—their feelings of powerlessness versus their sense of safety. The balance or imbalance may be articulated around notions of evil.

Sets of ideas are transmitted to all children as part of common knowledge of religion and understanding. This chapter shows how children are drawn into the religious life of a community. Children partake of ways of viewing the world. The emphasis is not on secrets: children are not excluded from knowledge. Indeed, it is striking how little is kept from children despite claims made for secret recipes and observations by elders of the ignorance of their children. The religious life of a community is an area of inclusion for children, rather than exclusion.

APPENDIX 1

BASED ON the 1982 census, plus projections, the Central Statistical Office (CSO) of the government of Zimbabwe estimated the 1989 population at nine million people. Those who speak chiShona predominate, forming about 75 percent of the population. Zezuru people, who speak a dialect of chiShona, form the largest cluster. An excerpt from *Progress Reports on Health and Development in Southern Africa,* 1989 (Fall/Winter): 12, gives pertinent statistics on Zimbabwe:

Infant Mortality Rate	76/1000 (a)
Population 1987	8.6 million (a)
Population 2000	12.5 million (a)
Annual Population Growth Rate	3 per cent (a)
Total Fertility	6.5 children per woman (a)
Literacy	66 percent (b)
Crude Birth Rate	42/1000 (c)
Life Expectancy	59 years (c)
Gross National Product per capita	US $620 per annum (c)
Population < 15 years	46 percent (a)

(a) Ministry of Health, Government of Zimbabwe, 1987
(b) Ministry of Education, Government of Zimbabwe, 1988
(c) *State of the World's Children, 1989,* United Nations Children's Fund, Geneva, 1989.

APPENDIX 2

THE STORY OF CHIHATA'S EMERGENCE AS A HEALER

CHIHATA IS the most renowned diviner-healer in her area. She was over eighty years old in 1982. She is small, slight, very wrinkled, and she wears thick glasses. Chihata often wears a khaki hat with her name and *Chiremba Mukuru* ("important herbalist") embroidered on it. She adorns herself with silver earrings, bracelets, and anklets. Born in Mozambique, she was brought to Rhodesia in the first decade of the century when she was about seven years old. The family settled in the Makota area.

Soon after arriving in the country Chihata fell ill and began to dream of flying and then dropping into the river. The dream recurred frequently. She told her parents the dream and they consulted diviners who said she would be "collected" (possessed) one day. They tied a *zango* (charm) around her neck to keep the spirits from possessing her, but it failed. She began to dream of plants and to heal. But, she says, she was a wild, naughty child and resented the idea of healing—the duty and the bother. She was paid in kind with chickens, flour, and bangles. When she refused to treat patients, her father would thrash her with a cane and bring her to the patient, in front of whom she would immediately become possessed.

To stop her being rude and naughty the spirits made her ill. At the age of about thirteen the *njuzu* (river) spirits decided to end her nonsense and make her treat willingly by taking her beneath the water. While she was fishing in the Magaba River with a friend, the spirits caused a whirlwind to pull her in, and they kept her for four days. Her friend called the family and her mother began to cry. She was quickly told to stop because if you cry for one taken by the *njuzu* they will never allow the person to return. Senior diviners were called and a ritual was held on the river bank. Drums were played and a female goat was thrown in the water. After four days one of the diviners, called Mutukumirwa, saw the child on a rock in the river. He swam to her and found beside her a small axe (*kano*), a shell-like white ornament (*ndoro*), and a cowrie-shell head band (*mbamba*).

Once out of the river she vomited fish and did not eat for two days. Then a *bira* (ritual feast) was held. Thereafter she treated conscientiously. She is the tenth person in her family to be possessed by a healing *shave*. She inherited it from her father's father, who had inherited it from his father's mother. Her father was also a diviner-healer and his *mudzimu* was passed on to him from his mother. Chihata's grandmother's possessions were given to her as a teenager to quieten the spirit that sought to possess her.

While under water Chihata learned a song. She sang it for me sometimes, once with her brother's wife, son, and grandchildren. It was eerily moving to hear her high, clear voice lead the others' voices and to see her body shake as she sat forward with her face in her hands. Here is the song:

Oh my! This spirit,
Oh my! This is my father's spirit.
Ho! Ho! Ha! I am called *Makuwerere:*[1] I have come.
Oh my! These drums are my father's,
It's Father, hey! I am *Makuwerere,* I have come.
He! He! I fell into the river.
Oh my! Oh my! This is my father's spirit,
It's Father, hey! I am *Makuwerere,* I will come.
He! He! Ya! Fellows, darkness has come
He! He! Ya! I am from Rukaya, I have come.
He! He! He! *Makuwerere hoye!*
It's me, yes, it's Chihata who has come, hey!
I will leave it to my child.

---

[1]*Makuwerere*—outstanding event, achievement, spectacle.

It's Father, fellows, this is Father here,
It's Father who gave me these things.
I will go to Magaba, I have come,
And so mother I have come,
I have left the world I have come,
It's me, Father, the widow—I have come.
He! He! Once I bury another child I will come.
This *shave* I have is my father's.
Four days I was under water,
Then I was rescued by other *chiremba.*
Now I am all alone.
These are my father's drums,
When I die I will leave behind poverty.
Haiye! Haiye! Hoye!

APPENDIX 3

THE FOLLOWING is Alec J. C. Pongweni's (1982, 96–8) free translation of the song "Chirizevha Chapera" by Thomas Mapfumo and the Acid Band.

Chirizevha chapera.
Hoihere mambo;
Chirizevha chapera
Hoihere baba;
Chirizevha chapera.

The fabric of rural society has been rended.
Oh Yes, Lord
Things have fallen apart,
There can be no doubt about that;
Mere anarchy is loosed upon the earth.

Hinga zvinonzwisa tsitsi mambo,
Ona zvinonzwisa tsitsi mambo,
Hinga zvinonzwisa tsitsi mambo.

This is a sad spectacle,
There's utter misery,
My heart melts to see these things.

Hoihere baba,
Chirizevha chapera;
Hoihere baba,
Chirizevha chapera;
Hoihere mambo,
Chirizevha chapera;
Hoihere baba,
Chirizevha chapera.

Our dear father,
Our communal culture has been dislocated.
Our dear father,
Our communal culture has been dislocated.

Chembere dzaikanga mudyakari, parizevha;
Harahwa dzaiveza mupinyi, parizevha

The old women cooking favorite dishes,
The old men carving beauty,

Mapfumo aichema.
Mheterwa dzaitsviriridzwa mumakura
parizevha.
Tuzukuru twaienda kumombe honde,
Parizevha.

Beating iron into spears,
The young whistling in the
 echoing bush.
The grandchildren herding
 cattle
All this pastoral existence is
 gone from the face of the
 earth.

Hoihere mambo,
Vaitamba chigendeya
Hoihere baba
Vaitamba chigendeya;
Hoihere baba
Vaitamba chinhundurwa,
Hoihere baba
Chirizevha chapera.

Yes, our people used to dance
 the joy dance
Yes, you can't believe it
But they used to
Yes, our people used to dance
 the joy dance
Yes, you can't believe it
But they used to.

Hondo inonzwisa tsitsi mambo,
Hondo inonzwisa tsitsi mambo iwe,
Hondo inonzwisa tsitsi mambo.

War unleashes suffering,
It opens the floodgates of hell,
To swallow the innocent.

Vamwe vakadimuka makumbo nayo,
Vamwe ndokufira ipapo mambo,
Vamwe ndokutsvira mudzimba iwe.
Vamwe vakatiza hondo kumusha.

Some of our people lost their
 limbs,
Others their life on the spot,
Some were roasted alive in
 their huts,
While the lucky found refuge in
 the towns.

Hinga zvinonzwisa tsitsi mambo.
Hinga zvinonzwisa tsitsi mambo iwe.
Hinga zvinonzwisa tsitsi mambo.
Hinga zvinonzwisa tsitsi mambo iwe,
Hondo inonzwisa tsitsi mambo.

It melts my heart to recount
 these things.
My song is a chronicle of sad
 events.
I cannot keep these happenings
 out of my mind,
They haunt me!

Vamwe vakadimuka makumbo nayo,
Vamwe ndokufira ipapo mambo,

Some of our people lost their
 limbs,

Vamwe ndokutsvira mudzimba iwe.
Vamwe vakatiza hondo kumusha iwe.

Others their life on the spot,
Some were roasted alive in
their huts,
While the lucky found refuge in
the towns.

Hondo inonzwisa tsitsi mambo.
Chirizevha chapera,
Hondo inonzwisa tsitsi mambo.

The war turns the world upside
down.
Communal life is now a tattered
fabric because of the war.

APPENDIX 4

GIVEN BELOW are three case studies of the killing of civilians by government forces. The first two are taken from Catholic Commission for Justice and Peace 1977.

KILLING OF THREE CHILDREN AND A TEACHER
AT KANDENGA SCHOOL, 18 APRIL 1977

A recent incident in which security forces killed three children and a teacher and wounded twelve other children is a tragic example of the gravity of the situation. In this case, as in many others, the version of the security forces differs substantially from the accounts given by the injured victims and other eye witnesses. Furthermore, it appears that an attempt was made to hide the matter from the public and the story never appeared in the official Security Force Headquarters communique and was only published in the newspapers eleven days after the incident occurred. There were also factual errors in the report. The school was misnamed Kandeya rather than Kandenga. Four children were reported dead rather than three, and no names or details were given of the dead or injured children.

The "contact tragedy," as it was termed by the newspapers, took place at 12:30 on the afternoon of 18 April at Kandenga School, which is about 10 km from the Sabi river in the Sabi Tribal Trust Land. According to the newspaper account, "Terrorists in this area are regarded by the security forces as being the most aggressive they are fighting."

The story, which first appeared in the 29 April edition of the *Rhodesia Herald,* quoted only a "security forces spokesman" and gave the following account. There had been several ambushes by "terrorists" in the vicinity of the school and on 18 April ten "terrorists" were sighted in the area. Five were seen moving through the bush and entering the school. According to the spokesman, "The terrorists rounded up the pupils and moved them out of the buildings to the centre of the school grounds." At this stage the ground patrol of the army called for assistance from the air force and five helicopters flew to the scene.

As the helicopters approached the school, some of the children and the "terrorists" rushed into one of the buildings while the others scattered to hiding places throughout the school compound. The security forces claim that there was no firing from the helicopters as they circled the school. (There are bullet holes in the roof of the school.)

The security forces allege that the "terrorists" opened fire on the ground forces, who returned it but aimed high to miss the children, which accounts for the bullet holes in the roof. When two of the "terrorists" ran from the building towards a hedgerow about 50 m away they were killed by a stop group of the security forces. Another two met the same fate when they also ran from the building in the same direction. The spokesman admitted that the guerrillas "did not use the children as a shield."

The stop groups north of the school then saw a movement in the grass about 100 m away. Security forces opened fire. According to the newspaper, "It was in that action that the four children were killed and others were injured." The spokesman explained that the children had run from the school building to take cover in the bush.

The teacher, Mr. Jackson Tachiona Maisiri, died in the building where the "terrorists" reportedly fled. "At some stage security forces' ground fire was directed at this particular building," was the vague explanation of the security forces spokesman.

Both the security forces spokesman and the schoolchildren agree that the contact lasted for a long time. "It went on for longer than the security forces would have liked," their spokesman said. "The reason was that there were schoolchildren in the grounds and the security forces made every effort not to involve them."

The fifth "terrorist" was reported to have escaped. The bodies of four "terrorists" and their weapons and personal equipment were alleged to have been recovered from the scene.

The children and the teachers tell an entirely different story. They steadfastly maintain that there were no guerillas at the school that morning. At 12:30 all the pupils were assembled in the school yard for dismissal when they saw helicopters circling overhead. The head teacher and school children ran towards the school gate (gate A) where two of the helicopters were landing outside the wire fence surrounding the compound. Three European soldiers got out with guns. Without any warning they shot into the group of children, killing three: Jenni Kandenga (grade 7), Zeketia Zvekure (grade 2), and Raphinos Zariro (aged 3 years). Others were injured, including: Nyevero Zariro (16 years) with a bullet grazing her shin; Grace Zariro (grade 7) with a bullet which passed through her right shoulder; James Kujinga (grade 1) with a bullet in his thigh above his knee; Sarah Mutsauri (grade 6) was also injured. All the above were taken to Buhera Hospital.

Janet Nyembe (grade 6) and Sarudzai Kandenga (grade 4) were both taken to Enkeldoorn Hospital with bullet wounds. Enos Kandenga was badly wounded and taken to Harare Hospital as was a teacher, Mr. Eddison Chivongodza, who was shot in the shoulder.

Two soldiers then went around the classrooms. Another teacher, Mr. Jackson Tachiona Maisiri, had hidden under some desks and was shot dead. Shots were fired through the roofs of the classroom from a helicopter circling overhead and a grenade was dropped from the helicopter near the latrine injuring teacher Muchina, who was hiding there.

On 2 May, the *Rhodesia Herald* carried an editorial on the incident entitled, "Tragic Event," expressing regret at the loss of young lives and questioning the attempt to hide the matter from the public.

It stated, "We believe that nothing was gained by failing to release details of the tragedy for ten days, and then only after inquiries from the newspapers. In the absence of any official news, rumour was given time to grow and spread. It is on unfortunate incidents like this that the enemies of Rhodesia feed. . . . It may be that details of the incident at Kandeya were not known to those responsible for keeping the public informed. But they most certainly ought to have been."

35 CIVILIANS KILLED AT DABWA AND 31 INJURED, 6 MAY 1977

Another "tragic event" took place the following month when 35 African civilians, including women and children, were killed and 31 others wounded at Dabwa kraal in the southern area of Ndangwa Tribal Trust Land. According to the *Rhodesia Herald,* this was the worst reported incident of civilian deaths since September 1976, when more than 30 were killed.

Those dead at Dabwa included sixteen women, twelve children and seven men. They were gathered in the kraal with approximately 200 others when the shooting took place at about 9:30 Friday night, 6 May.

The incident was reported briefly in the official security forces communique of 9 May and the newspaper account of 10 May was based on evidence given by Superintendent Jim Carse of the special branch in charge of the Criminal Investigation Division in the Chiredzi area. According to Supt. Carse, the civilians were killed in crossfire between about nine "terrorists" and fifteen members of the security force who were on a "normal follow-up operation."

The contact followed the robbery of two buses in the area. "The security forces on the ground entered the kraal as a result of information they received," explained Supt. Carse. "As they entered the kraal area it was obvious to them that a meeting was in progress . . . and it was obvious to the African members of the patrol that it was a terrorist who was addressing the meeting. They were close enough to hear the terrorist."

At this point, a lone sentry is reported to have opened fire on the security forces. "After the terrorists opened fire the security forces did the same thing," reported Supt. Carse. "Panic ensued with people running everywhere. After seven minutes the security forces ceased fire."

Only one "terrorist" is reported to have been killed in the operation and there were no casualties among the security forces. According to the security forces communique, several "terrorists" were wounded and "quantities of communist arms and equipment were found at the scene."

While Supt. Carse admitted that the killing of civilians was an "unfortunate setback," he placed the blame on the victims. "I think the locals knew they had done wrong by allowing the terrorists to come into the area and call a meeting," he said. Shortly before blaming the villagers, however, the Supt. himself stated, "They know they have got to attend these meetings, otherwise the terrorists may come back and kill them."

The incident had greatly upset the security forces according to Lieutenant-Colonel Cedric French. "They don't like to see innocent civilians killed whatever the circumstances," he said.

An editorial in the *Rhodesia Herald* of 11 May entitled "Victims of War" commented on the event, observing that "such tragedies are unfortunately inevitable in fighting of this nature." It continued, "The security forces have given a frank account of the events that led to the shooting. There is no reason to disbelieve it. After all, when bullets and people start to fly on a dark night who can say who is friend or foe, let alone civilian?"

The security forces also defended the operation, saying that they had "no alternative but to open fire." Though not actually present during the operation, Supt. Carse said, "I am completely satisfied that they acted as I would have if I had been there. . . . I cannot see us altering instructions to security forces to cease firing if they are being fired at by terrorists." June 1977.

22 DIE IN VILLAGE ATTACK

Twenty-two people—all but three of them women and children—died when security forces carried out a ground and air attack on a village early on Saturday afternoon. One of the dead was a terrorist.

The security forces were in the area after a report that six terrorists had been seen on a hill feature close to the village. According to a relative of one of the dead women, the terrorists scattered when security force aircraft crossed the feature.

At least one of the terrorists, he said, ran to the village. He mingled with the villagers outside the home of Mr Ben Mashonganyika. As the security forces approached, he entered a kitchen to one side of the house. It was in the kitchen that eleven of the latest victims of the bush war died. Another two died outside the house and nine more burned to death in a hut hit by security forces' fire a few metres away.

The village is about 12 km from the Salisbury boundary, in a tribal trust land. Eyewitnesses said mixed sticks of white and black security forces were used in the operation. In addition to the 22 who died, four villagers were injured. A number of buildings were damaged during the action. One of the villagers, Mr Jairos Nyakudya (40), said the operation started some time after noon.

"It was quite unexpected," he said. "We heard the planes and then there was this loud thump, and people started running in all directions in a panic. Then we saw the security forces. They aimed their fire at the kitchen."

It was only last night, when one of the relatives spoke to journalists in Salisbury, that it became apparent that there was a terrorist presence in the village. Earlier in the day, the villagers had denied the fact.

It is understood security forces recovered an assault rifle of communist origin from the scene. The incident was confirmed in an official communique issued late last night. The military command said a search of the village by the security forces also revealed loaded magazines, a mortar bomb and a quantity of smallarms ammunition of communist origin. The command said the armed terrorists had been sighted with a group of civilians.

"This group scattered on the approach of the security forces and fire was directed by the terrorists at the security forces," the communique stated. "Terrorists were seen, with others of the group, to run into a nearby village." The communique said ammunition was heard to explode within the hut that caught fire, from which nine unidentified bodies were later recovered.

It was also reported that on Friday night a communist grenade was thrown into the bar of a hotel in a tribal trust land north-west of Salisbury. It exploded among the civilians in the bar, injuring nine men, two of them seriously.

Security forces have killed eight more terrorists.

Defence reporter Chris Reynolds
Rhodesia Herald, 12 June 1978

APPENDIX 5

A BINGA schoolboy wrote the following account of his experiences of violence from both sides during the war:

IT WAS A HARD-WON FREEDOM

Most areas suffered terribly during the war. Many people lost property at irreplaceable expense.

Like other areas in Zimbabwe, Kariyangwe was subject to the plundering and other scandalous activities of the war. The devil perpetually showed his ugly face. Life had become too short for everybody. Things had become so bad at one time that I thought of absconding from Zimbabwe and losing myself in the vast world. However, this idea could not materialise as it was only contained in the heart of a tortured soul. Physical contact with any other people or relatives in other areas was cut off.

One worried about life alone and nothing else. Day after day reports of deaths, torment or arrests of civilian people by either belligerent parties was common news. There was no side better than the other in any practical sense. People suffered the same troubles from either side, the guerrilla forces and the Rhodesian African Rifle forces, as they were called.

Of the worst that befell me during the struggle, there was one terrible incident which ever floods my mind and takes precedence whenever I try to review the troubles. This was the day when the man who was the chairman of a secret organisation responsible for the food supplies and information for the guerrillas was killed and his home set on fire. This man was only responsible for a certain portion of Kariyangwe, called Lubu. His name was Zumanana Mudimba. He was quite a famous and important man. During the years of drought he could sell grain to those who had nothing in their granaries.

Whenever the guerrillas entered Lubu, they had to be reported to Mr Mudimba, so that he could prepare for their needs, if any. Usually the only thing that they needed was food. These were the disciplined and honest forces of 1977 and early 1978.

Towards the end of 1978 and early 1979, the situation suddenly changed. Trouble came to the crunch; the old adage, "Each man for himself but God for us all," involuntarily came into full use. Brother fought against brother in the bush, father against son, and so forth. They hunted one another down in the struggle for life and death.

The guerrillas would come to Mr Mudimba and ask for food. As time dragged on, the guerrillas increased in number; more and more of them were young and not fully experienced, undisciplined in manner. Their attitude towards civilians was abominable. Now they could not do as they used to do in the early days, and act with restraint. They turned Mr Mudimba's home into a centre for their enjoyment and corruption. This was when I truly saw corruption. The guerrillas could come to Mr Mudimba's home in their numbers and order goats, chickens or an ox to be slaughtered. More than this, they sent for girls to prepare their meals; at night these girls turned into their wives. The elders knew this; they hated the whole concept but they were powerless to do anything to correct the situation. But now, remember, above all the guerrillas had put civilians in a very precarious position. It was obvious that they could not keep the Rhodesian forces from knowing about this; it would leak somehow.

The guerrillas violated the governing social code and were doing the most preposterous things, quite unimaginable. Sleeping around with women publicly in any society is a social taboo; nature itself does not allow it. But the guerrillas had made it a common item on the market. They enjoyed themselves deep into the night with girls, whilst boys were deployed in the bush around the home as guards, so that they would warn the guerrillas if enemies came. Unfortunately I was one of those boys who did this duty. Now, being a guard, un-armed, meant that one had to keep awake until around four o'clock, when they departed on patrol to far places. Life had really become uncertain for boys and girls, and I was more than prepared to run away with them one day and come back with my own gun.

Somehow, as I have already said, the news that the guerrillas had an established centre where they enjoyed themselves during the night got into the hands of the Rhodesian forces at the "keep" or protected camp, about 8 km from Kariyangwe Mission. They decided to come in broad daylight rather than at night, when the guerrillas were available. This alone was quite indicative of their aim. Of course: to deal with the civilians. Their number again made one doubt if anyone had remained at their camp. The strategy was that they must make sure that the people were dealt with thoroughly. The first two went straight to Mr Mudimba's village to prevent him from running away. The rest drove the multitudes of people collected from their homes towards Mr Mudimba's village. The devil had descended on Lubu and I could almost see him approach.

"Things must be done to our satisfaction, guys," cried the white commander, whose cruelty seemed congenital rather than acquired. His face alone was dangerous to look at. His stern eyes, which almost filled his jaded face, had a stinging look.

Darkness fell upon me in broad daylight. I was enveloped by an atmosphere of terrible fear. There was total and horrendous violence. The Rhodesian forces probed into the huts of the people and scattered everything. Mealie-meal was their first target. They scattered it in the air, and the sky and earth was filmed over by the white dust of mealie-meal. As a result, they felt, the guerrillas would starve when they came back.

The fierce appearance and bullying ways of the Rhodesian forces made people move their feet at unimagined speed, and we found ourselves gathered at Mr Mudimba's home in an extremely short time. The commander told people that he and his colleagues were going to demonstrate that they had purposely remained patient with the ordinary people but, such patience was going to end.

No one coughed; everyone waited for what would follow. For me it was as if the world had come to an end. I had already imagined myself dead and appearing before God on judgement day.

Things had to be done as the commander had ordered. Torture was experienced at its extreme. Women were ordered to bring buckets full of water. A confused stampede prevailed; questions were asked but no answer was listened to. Whether one answered or kept quiet, it was all the same because one would still receive a hard blow. They did not care what they used to hit with; anything that was to hand could be used. If one was found to be a little stubborn, they held him up by the legs head downward and lowered him into a bucket full of water, holding him like that as long as they wished. He would struggle and struggle, cry as much as possible; but to them that was amusement, and they laughed.

The work was done now—but remember, they had not yet touched Mr Mudimba. Many people lay convincingly unconscious; some were even bleeding to death. It was a horrible scene. I was lucky because I was not in such a serious position but was given a hard blow which dazed me and I found myself lying prostrate on the ground after a few minutes.

The people were then told to move into a small clearing that was in front of the chairman's home. Those who had some little strength to use stood and squatted there. A chair was brought for the chairman, and he was made to sit before his people.

"Now talk to your people as you always do," said one of the soldiers, "or else we shoot you straight away." Bravely, the chairman stood up and told the soldier that he had nothing to say and he had never held any meeting before; if they wanted to kill him they could do so. Before he actually finished the words the bang of the gun was heard and the chairman collapsed to the ground before his people. The bullet had gone right through his chest. His wife came from the bush where she was hiding herself from the horrible scene, and leaped forward to nurse her husband. As she bent down in grief over the cold recumbent figure, she received a hard kick on the backside from the soldier who was standing nearby. "You wife of the devil!" was his comment. The poor woman staggered once and hit the ground head-first with a loud thud.

Things did not end here. Still the commander, with his war-like voice, dry and croaky, ordered his boys to set the *ngazis* [granaries] on fire. Only those which contained grain had to be set on fire. Within two minutes the boys had finished their work and from each *ngazi* emanated a flame which soon grew to a frightening blaze. The smoke from burning grain obscured the sunlight and cast a darkish shadow over the bleak land.

I was turned to stone, cold and breathless. I felt something gnawing at my knees, and something drumming in my ears. Things had changed from reality to nightmare. I began to tremble uncontrollably. People's faces were dry and vacant. Each one stood where he had stood when he arrived, and never moved an inch.

When they returned to the camp, the soldiers took with them four men, ten girls and some boys. There these people experienced great torture, such that they ended up saying any untrue thing, hoping that it would save them from such heavy affliction.

The horrific experiences of that day left me weak. Whenever I reviewed the scene in my mind, I experienced the same drumming and throbbing of my heart. The same loathing of the experience pervaded my body like an aching wound, until I knew it was impossible to face life in that way. I also needed to hold a gun—but by then it was too late for any action.

APPENDIX 6

Below I reprint an extract from Bruce Moore-King (1988, 14-20):

There is no question of post-mortems in a war situation. . . . As in any war situation, there are occasions when seemingly innocent persons become enmeshed in the effective prosecution of operations. [Official Rhodesian spokesman, 11 June 1976]

This is the way it was.

A foot patrol moves from a group of small hills, bright light and long shadows in the early dawn.

They are six, young men, not zealots, not idealists, not even exceptional soldiers, just a patrol, a tracking group, army code name "sparrows," call sign "four one bravo." They have been on spoor three days, chasing a group of four, one pair of Bata Super Pro's, two chevroned pairs of boots, one pair of feet, bare for the last two days.

At last light the day before, the tracks brought them within sight of the small kraal before them, so they moved quietly to the top of a hill, hid carefully and watched through the night.

Nothing.

From the spoor, they were about five hours behind the group. Now they must add the hours of the past night.

Over the last three days, they have learnt about the group, survivors from an original group of seven that had been in contact with a Grey's Scouts patrol.

They know what weapons they are carrying—one RPD, one SKS, two AKs—they know at least one is slightly wounded, that they are not carrying packs, only webbing, and one of them has abandoned his footwear—also Bata, but light tennis shoes—because the sole of one was splitting badly.

They have gathered all this information—excepting the abandonment of the shoes—from people they have met over the last three days.

They do not know where the group is heading.

Moving carefully around the kraal, they ignore the people watching fearfully from the huts, and circle the entire kraal area, checking paths and fields for spoor.

Nothing.

They circle once more, a wider diameter, feeling exposed and nervous.

Nothing.

They move into the kraal.

The three people are old. A man, two wives.

Their huts are poor, sparse, drab—highlighting the newness of gifts, his son, who is working in Salisbury, the old man says—he has the name of the company—has brought them:

A cheap transistor radio—Supersonic.

A set of enamelled cooking pots, vivid colours on white—Treger products.

A bottle of cane spirit—Mainstay—nearly empty.

Two lengths of bright cloth—for the wives.

New blankets.

And a grandson, three or four years old, wide-eyed and trembling behind a tightly grasped skirt.

No, he's not seen any terrorists, he hasn't seen anyone except his sister's husband's uncle who came to borrow an axe two weeks ago and hasn't yet returned it, which is a hell of a nuisance, because they're having to use a blunt, worn-out old one to cut firewood and, at his age, it's no joke, because his arthritis . . .

The women are told to go into one of the huts with the child.

The patrol leader, a corporal, hand signals to his spread-out men, and, with the old man, they move away from the huts, about two hundred yards, into the thick bush, where they don't feel so exposed.

The interrogation begins.

Twenty minutes later, the old man's eyes are swelling rapidly, blood is drying beneath his nose, his lips are split, remaining few teeth dyed red, he has urinated into his tattered trousers, and his back is a smouldering agony of fire from the kidney punches.

No he's not seen any terrorists recently, only once, months ago, he saw a group of armed men while he was out checking snares, but he was scared and hid although he remembers exactly where he saw them if the Lords, the white masters, want to go. . . . No, he didn't see any last night, No . . . No . . . No . . . No . . . No.

Gravel is mixed with the drying blood, red paste, a clown's overdone make-up, on a swollen caricature of a face.

The corporal thinks for a minute. He knows the old man won't talk.

The wives?

No. Well, maybe.

But, more likely . . .

He calls two of his men over, sends them for the grandchild and a bucket of water.

He watches his grandson twisting and whipping, arching, fighting to break the grip on his ankles, avoid the bucket below him. He hears the child's screams disappear into gurgles and bubbles of air in the bucket.

Again.

The question.

Again.

The child lies on the ground, writhing, spewing water.

The corporal picks him up by the ankles, tightly, countering the tremendous strength the little body can generate.

Again.

The question.

The boy's struggles are weaker.

Again . . .

Yes. Yes. He will tell them, he will talk.

The old man would rather die than cause his grandson harm. He talks.

"How many?"

Describe their weapons, their clothes.

What did they tell him?

"Where are they going?"

"WHERE ARE THEY GOING?"

Hands on the boys ankles.

He talks.

They repeat the questions, trying to catch him out in a lie.

Again.

Again.

"WHERE ARE THEY GOING?"

"WHY?"

"Yes. Yes." He overheard them talking while his wife was preparing food.

"Yes. Yes. Yes. Yes."

The corporal reaches for the radio.

A helicopter picks them up.

Yes, the information ties in with other bits of knowledge, gathered here and there.

A hill.

A meeting.

A big meeting.

Numbers are thrown around, thirty, forty, a hundred.

A machine speeds into motion.

Stop Groups.

Fire Force.

Air Strike.

Helicopters hammer frantically in the dawn light. Groups of soldiers sprint towards the base of a hill, rapid darts of movement, sliding into the shelter of rocks and trees.

On the hill, they realise . . . they are surrounded.

The smell of hot rifles, clatter of empty magazines on granite.

Sinking coldness on the hill as the thunder of jets rolls over the horizon.

Ripping explosion of cannon shells.

Shrill greeting of shrapnel.

Flickering trails of fiery light, then the rockets hit.

Slippery red fingers refusing to fit a fresh magazine.

Blood on stones . . .

They kill seven, capture five.

Six weeks later the corporal makes acting sergeant.

Six weeks later the grandson has been sent back to his parents.

Six weeks later the old man and his wives are locked in a hut and burnt to death.

It is a war of terror.

On both sides.

A thousand years and a million miles later, the corporal wonders what it was like for the old man and his wives.

Those last six weeks.

Just waiting.

APPENDIX 7

EXTRACTS FROM Catholic Commission for Justice and Peace, 1977.

PROTECTED VILLAGES ON THE INCREASE

At the last count (30 May) there were approximately 203 protected villages in Rhodesia, housing more than half a million people. These figures from informed sources on the spot are double the official government estimates of 250,000, or "a twelfth of the total tribal population."

The figures continue to climb as the government steps up its programme to establish protected villages in almost all operational areas. During the past rainy season (March) more than 100 new villages were established which would involve about 20,000 people according to the government's estimates of 2,000 people per village.

Nineteen tribal trust lands in Mashonaland and Manicaland are already affected, and two in Victoria Province. The people in the Wankie area of Matabeleland have also been told they are to be moved into PVs. Chiweshe TTL, just 45 miles north of Salisbury, where the first village was established in 1974, continues to have the highest village population with 120,000 people living in 21 villages.

It is difficult to get accurate figures of the villages, not only because they are going up so fast, but because they also come down just as quickly. They are popular targets for the guerrillas who cut the fences, liberate the people inside and burn down the huts. At the end of May the Provincial Commissioner for Internal Affairs, Mr Geoffrey Henson, admitted that since the beginning of the year there had been 70 guerrilla attacks on the villages. This is probably an underestimate.

The guerrillas have also played havoc on the village administration by attacking personnel of the Ministry of Internal Affairs who are responsible for running the villages. On 1 July, the Minister, Mr Jack Mussett, stated in Parliament that his department had suffered high casualties with 114 killed, 25 missing or abducted and 243 wounded. He interpreted this to mean that the villages were successfully disturbing the guerrillas and said, "protected villages are proving to be a thorn in the side of the enemy."

On 30 June Mr Mussett presented a policy statement on Internal Affairs in which he reiterated the government's plan of constructing protected villages. "As part of the Defence Plan," he said, "it was decided at national level to re-settle the African people of certain areas in protected villages. This has been done, firstly, to provide protection to the African civilian population from the terrorist onslaught, and secondly, to deprive the terrorists of their sources of food, shelter, information and recruits. . . . I will not try to pretend that the exercise has been without hardship or difficulties for the African men, women and children involved. It is a tremendous upheaval for any person to have to leave his or her home and to change from a traditional easy-going rural way of life to an urban type of existence with the constraints imposed by the needs of security. However, these temporary disadvantages must be balanced against the overriding advantage of being able to live in comparative safety. . . ."

The people affected do not think much of this advantage. Few have anything to fear from the guerrillas and feel no need to be "protected" from them. They are still in danger from the security forces and can be submitted to interrogation which includes torture and beating. There have been many cases of rape in the "keeps," as the villages are called locally, and District Assistants are known to confiscate the passes (*situpas*) of the women which allow them to move in and out of the village, and to force the women to sleep with them in order to retrieve their passes.

The "urban type of existence" mentioned consists of a small amount of space (often 15 square metres per family), lack of sanitary facilities, clean water and sufficient food. People must build new houses from whatever they can salvage from their former dwellings and receive no compensation for the property they lose. Families are moved up to five kilometres from their fields and are often unable to produce enough to feed themselves. Their cattle are kept outside the village and are frequently stolen. The education of their children is interrupted and sometimes terminated for good (47 schools have been closed because the population was moved into protected villages). The people are kept behind fences almost like prisoners and must call out their numbers and be registered when entering and leaving the village. . . .

Almost every week there is a feature story in the paper showing the success of a particular village and painting them in a very positive light. People on the spot give a different picture. "People have lost all hope," reported an official of the Salisbury Archdiocese who visited the Mtoko area in July where he saw people living out in the cold because their former houses had been burnt by the army and they were still building their new houses. Some people have had to move three times. A doctor from one area reported that the people do not come for treatment when they are sick. "They say they may as well die than live in such hell," the doctor said. . . .

A report from the Mtoko area in May stated, "The prime need of the people at the moment is blankets and this will be the prime need for at least the next three months. When winter comes to an end so will the food and from August onwards the prime need will be mealie-meal." A report from the Umtali Diocese in April states, "Already people are hungry in the protected villages and the situation food-wise is certain to deteriorate. Food and property were moved during the rains which were unusually severe this year. Much of the food is rotting. No ploughing was done as the people had to transport everything themselves and also to build huts."

Another report from Dande TTL in the north says, "Aid of any kind is most urgently needed for Mabomo and Chapoto. Mabomo was resettled in the bush without clinic, school, stores, post offices, etc. No cattle. Chapoto is cut from the outside world through war activities. Ganano is in a similar position. . . . Malaria is rampant. Villages west of the Utete river are not allowed to have any cattle because of tse-tse fly." From Chiweshe a report states, "Most desperate need of the people is safe sanitary facilities. Insufficient and polluted water poses a related problem to health and Chiweshe has been noted for the incidence of typhoid in the past."

More than half a million people have been forced to live in such difficult conditions and to create new lives from nothing. The real irony is that in many areas the guerrillas move in and out of villages freely. This has been confirmed by many people who say that the guerrillas either make friends with the DAs or threaten them. If the villages fail to cut off the guerrillas from the local population, what purpose do they serve except to make life miserable for their inhabitants?

APPENDIX 8

THE SUNDAY newspaper with the largest circulation in the country printed the following article based on medical practitioners' warnings of deteriorating health conditions during the war.

WAR SPREADS NEW WAVE OF DISEASES

A warning that dangerous infectious diseases and widespread epidemics could occur because of the war was given yesterday by the Rhodesian Medical Association executive council, representing about 400 doctors all over Rhodesia.

The president, Dr Paul Fehrsen, said that diseases such as sleeping sickness and rabies, which had previously been eradicated, were now being reported with increasing frequency.

The RMA executive had reviewed the effect of the war on the health of the people of Rhodesia, it said in a statement.

"If hostilities continue, epidemics and disease will become widespread in cities, towns and rural areas throughout Rhodesia." Listing seven points, the statement said:

Many small hospitals and clinics have closed, leaving millions of people without access to health facilities.

Many monthly maternal and child health facilities have been closed in different parts of every district.

This means that mothers cannot obtain advice about health matters, there are no accessible ante-natal or family planning facilities and children cannot be immunised against measles, diphtheria, whooping cough, tetanus, poliomyelitis and tuberculosis.

A number of children susceptible to these dangerous infectious diseases are growing up unimmunised.

Malnutrition among adults and children is increasing and is widespread in areas where stores have been closed and travel is dangerous.

Malaria, bilharzia and other endemic disease control programmes are curtailed and much of the ground gained over the years is being lost.

Most rural schools are closed.

Veterinary control programmes are being affected and tick-borne diseases have killed thousands of cattle belonging to Africans. Foot-and-mouth disease in one area means that cattle cannot be sold. Measures against rabies, tsetse fly and locusts are curtailed.

The routine of village life has been disrupted so that normal chores cannot be completed within curfew hours and every night is a time of anxiety and danger, the statement said.

"The tending of crops and cattle is neglected and there is an atmosphere of hopelessness in many villages."

The statement concluded: "As the tempo of the war increases, there is more brutality and ever increasing misery and hardship."

Dr Fehrsen said the Rhodesian Medical Association believed it necessary to present these facts to all the people of Rhodesia.

Sunday Mail, 28 January 1979

APPENDIX 9

THE FOLLOWING are accounts of one of the most well-known incidents when children were recruited and taken outside Rhodesia. They include press reports, and the account of one of the school teachers who accompanied the children on their journey.

PRESS REPORTS

TERRORISTS GRAB 400 AT MISSION
GUNPOINT MARCH FOR CHILDREN

by Chris Reynolds at Manama Mission (Botswana border)

A group of four terrorists burst into this isolated mission on Sunday night and forced 400 youngsters at gunpoint to leave their prayer meeting.

The youngsters, aged between 12 and 21, had just returned to school. The terrorists said they were from Zapu—Mr Joshua Nkomo's banned political organisation. They said they were taking them to Botswana as "army recruits."

Mr Nkomo was educated only a few kilometres from here. The young Africans included many girls. From the assembly hall where they were in prayer the youngsters were taken to a play area. The terrorists told them they would run—all the way to Botswana.

The scene in the play area yesterday was a sad reminder of the worst case of abduction since the St Albert's mission incident north of Centenary in 1973, when 250 children were taken by terrorists to Mozambique. School uniforms lay abandoned. So did shoes and food and hats and school books. A Bible lay open on the rain-soaked play area. The inscription, from 2nd Timothy, read:

"For I am already on the point of being sacrificed. The time of my departure has come."

The Bible belonged to a child of 15. Today, she is somewhere in Botswana. Her parents do not know it yet. Security forces have been able to contact only a few relatives so far. One mother, crying unashamedly, said here yesterday: "I feel tremendous pain." She has lost a boy of 14.

This is not the first time Zapu terrorists have come into this area to obtain recruits this year. About ten days ago they went into a beer garden near here and rounded up 185 men and women and took them to Botswana.

In this latest incident, 17 pupils managed to hide from the terrorists. Five more escaped after they crossed the Sashe River into Botswana. One of these, a young man, said yesterday: "They told us we would get better education in Botswana. They took us away at gunpoint. They said they would kill us if we tried to run away."

The young man, well-spoken, is 21. Before this incident he had read about terrorists only in the newspapers. "I did not believe them," he said. "Now I have first-hand knowledge. Once in Botswana I hid in the bush and at the first opportunity I escaped."

He said pupils were ordered out of assembly at gun-point as the school bell was ringing. At that point the headmaster was in his house preparing the school fees for banking—a total of $13,000. He has been at the mission school for six years. "I was in my office when the terrorists arrived," he said. "An armed man came in and said, 'Old man, I want money.'" The headmaster related how he opened a safe and took out $10. "The man had a rifle that was different to those carried by the security forces," he said. "He told me, 'Rubbish.' He said I had to tell him where the real money was or he would kill me. He said he was Zapu. I told him the money for the school fees was at my house. I said I would go with them instead of the children." But the terrorists gave him one of their AK bullets "as evidence they had been at the mission" and told him not to report the incident until the following day.

As the children were marched away from the mission one of the evangelical missionaries arrived at the gates in his car. The terrorists ordered him out at gunpoint. He left his child in the back of the vehicle. The terrorists made him join the children, and walk and run for three and a half hours. The terrorists then robbed a bottle store, and he escaped. Why did he leave the children, some of whom had fainted on the forced march? "I thought I was being forced into something I did not believe in," he said. The mission matron rescued his child from his car. She was one of the silent heroes. For she also guided three boys and two girls to the safety of her house from the terrorists. "I am just worried and confused," she said yesterday. "I pray the children will be all right."

Rhodesia Herald, 1 February 1977

The *Rhodesia Herald* carried stories on 2nd, 4th and 5th February 1977 on the diplomatic and parliamentary maneuverings, by the Smith and British governments, to repatriate the children from Botswana through the Red Cross. Some 112 parents of the children (230 boys and 170 girls) were taken to Francistown to see if the children would return. Only a few did so. The reports continued.

MANAMA CHILDREN FLY TO ZAMBIA

Report from Lusaka

More than 100 schoolgirls who left the Manama Mission in southwestern Rhodesia and crossed into Botswana last week were flown here aboard a chartered Swaziland aircraft yesterday.

On Sunday, 333 of the 384 mission students refused to return to Rhodesia with their parents who went to Francistown to fetch them, reports Iana-AP.

After the girls arrived here yesterday they were whisked off under tight security to Makeni refugee camp south of the city. When all the students arrive in Zambia they will be moved from the Makeni camp to terrorist bases in Mozambique, where they will be trained by cadres in the Zimbabwe People's Army, which is the military arm of the Patriotic Front coalition between Mr Robert Mugabe's Zanu and Mr Joshua Nkomo's Zapu organisations (both banned in Rhodesia). In a statement issued in Lusaka, Zapu said the Manama Mission students were joining the "liberation struggle" to topple the Rhodesian Government. Our London Bureau says that the British Government has still not taken up a firm position on whether or not it accepts responsibility for those of the children who are minors. Repeated questioning of the Foreign and Commonwealth office elicited no more than the statement that there was a great deal of confusion still over the exact situation at Francistown and that a full report had not yet been received from the British diplomat, Mr P. Raftery, who went to the camp in which the children have been housed.

The Centre Party said last night it was deplorable that the British and Botswana Governments appeared to have ignored the fundamental principle, not only of European, but of African customary law, that minor children are subject to the control and guardianship of their parents.

"At the very least those minor children, whose parents, or their representatives, went to Botswana to reclaim them should have been released to their parents' custody without any question, whatever the children's stated wishes may have been," said a statement.

Rhodesia Herald, 9 February 1977

CHILDREN SAFE

Zambia Africa News Service, Lusaka

The Zambian Government has denied the reported execution of Rhodesian schoolchildren who went to Zambia to join the terrorists.

The Ministry of Home Affairs said there was "absolutely no truth" in the reports in foreign newspapers that 15 of the children from a Rhodesian mission school who had gone to Zambia through Botswana had been murdered by Zapu because they insisted on joining the rival Zanu (both organisations are banned in Rhodesia).

A spokesman for the Ministry said the Zambian Government

wished to assure parents of children who had chosen to fight with the Rhodesian "guerrillas" that none had been killed by "freedom fighters" of either Zapu or Zanu.

The Government, he said, was "appalled and disgusted" by the reports and intended immediately to track down the originators who would be "mercilessly punished."

Sunday Mail, 6 March 1977

A SCHOOLTEACHER'S ACCOUNT

Paulus Matjaka, a teacher at Manama Mission School at the time, wrote of the incident in *So That Our Youngsters Will Know*, J. Z. Moyo Social History Project (Harare: Baobab, forthcoming):

On Sunday I left my home earlier than usual to return to Manama. My departure was so sudden that I left half a bottle of beer standing in the sitting room. I drove to Manama, stopping briefly in the village at Bottle Store No. 8. Then for some reasons I left my drink as I had done at home, and went to the school. Just as I entered, there were guerrillas rounding up the school. There was stampeding as the students ran here and there. I joined them, with almost all the students.

We started about 5:30 or 6:00 P.M. from Manama. Before sunrise we were crossing the Shashi, the last person was actually coming out of the river as the sun rose. We heard a spotter plane, and were told to take cover. There was much confusion. The spotter was flying along the river, and had clearly seen our footmarks in the sand. It returned, then cruised ahead of us to show we had been seen. The guerrillas were on the point of deciding to shoot down the spotter. But they didn't. We reached Gobazhango, this time followed by helicopters. Twice we had to take cover because they were right above our heads. We were really vulnerable in our red school uniforms.

At Gobazhango it was decided to cook food for us. Fortunately there was a cattle sale and we could mix with the crowds, but later people dispersed. We were really obvious. At 4:00 P.M. we were told to go where food had been prepared for us. It was an open area. He-

licopters came and started terrorising us—they flew so low that they
caused a dust storm, and the children were stampeding in every direction. I felt so convinced they were going to kill us, I said let's just look
at the colour of a bomb, before we die . . . but they did not shoot or
bomb us at all. They didn't want to kill schoolchildren when they
could gain some favour with the parents. (In fact they later issued
quick passports to parents to come to Francistown in Botswana.)

We ate and slept in the bush. Now the problem became discipline.
There was a problem of stress. The children started wanting each
other, until with so many running for help to the adults we felt sunk
by this problem. In fact, many students and even some teachers had
dropped out by this time, but I refused to leave the children.

After 12:00 midnight there was a flare. An aeroplane was flying over
us, and it was as clear as if it was daytime, we could see into each
other's faces. Then we saw clouds starting to build up. Then, one of the
freedom fighters, a guerrilla called Bob, came to us and told us we were
stupid. How could we remain after a plane had passed over us? We
were told to move. He led us. Heavy rain started falling. There were
thorny bushes, darkness, and now it was muddy. We lost our shoes.
(We had raided a store before leaving for food and clothing. . . .)
Children got caught in the thorns, and we were constantly calling:
"Matjaka! Matjaka! I can't move!" We pulled them out, tearing clothes
and often leaving the clothes behind caught in the thorns. It didn't
matter to anyone if they were half-naked.

Bob had arranged with the chief for us to sleep in the school buildings so we would not be seen. But that night there were still children
screaming. The following morning we woke up to find ourselves completely surrounded by the Botswana Army. They were fully equipped
for a war in our defence. The chief had decided to call for them, and
had telephoned. They were ready to shoot any planes coming from
Rhodesia, but no more came. Someone had brought a radio from
Halisupi and we heard about the whole incident involving us—the
Rhodesians said: "The Botswana Army seems to be provoking a fight!"
It was arranged for us to be ferried away by Botswana lorries. The
youngest boys and girls went first, then the older girls, then the older
boys and us. We were escorted by the Botswana Army. At Gubunom,
we were fed by the United Nations. Two days later we were ferried to

Selibe Phikwe. There we were accommodated for a day in the prison, where we met Zimbabwean prisoners. Then we carried on to Francistown, in very rainy weather. Real adventure for those who wanted that. . . .

In Francistown there were all sorts of happenings. One night, shootings caused a lot of confusion. We thought Rhodesian forces were on the other side of the river from the kopje that overlooks the town. Both the guerrillas and Botswana Army fired back. There were no casualties. Later on a guerrilla let off his rifle, and when the Botswana Army started firing back, we realised our mistake.

There were two camps, one for ZANU and one for ZAPU. Our relations were tense, especially among the youth. The United Nations came, and also some Botswana VIPs, to talk and offer comfort. Rhodesia had asked Botswana to keep us there, so that parents could collect their children. Buses of parents came. They parked away from the camp, and the children were taken in groups. As for me, three times I was asked by the parents to come and talk at the meeting place. First it was a cousin who was sent to ask me. He thought I was being stupid. The second was the Headmaster of Manama. The third who came to ask me was another relative. Each time, I refused. It was not relatives who should be seen by the people who had come to Francistown, but the children.

Chartered planes were then arranged to take us to Zambia. It took 8 or 9 days to be processed. We were feeling vulnerable, we could be bombarded by the Rhodesian forces. But maybe the war was not yet hot enough—they never came, and also it was schoolchildren who had been abducted. Out of the children, the radical ones were enjoying the excitement, I would say about 90 per cent of them. Those who were unhappy, the majority of them had their chance to go back when the parents came.

APPENDIX 10

WITCH-HUNTER'S REIGN OF TERROR IN MREWA

by Giles Kuimba

MORE THAN 250 alleged witches, spirits (*vadzimu*) and evil forces (*mashave*) were "smelt out" from among about 3,000 people at a ceremony at Msami near St Paul's Mission in Mrewa district yesterday afternoon.

The ceremony was part of a witch-hunting wave that is sweeping the district. Riding the wave is self-proclaimed spirit medium from Malawi, Mr Size Kapara Chikanga, who has taken the area by storm. He claims he can "smell out" witches, wizards, evil spirits, curses, spells, and cure all types of illness.

Mr Chikanga, who said he came from the Dedza district of Malawi, showed a *Sunday Mail* team an assortment of witchcraft paraphernalia which he said had been brought with him by "repentant and cured witches." On show were greasy calabashes, animal horns and bottles full of black concoctions which he said were the tools of the witchcraft trade. Among them was a flywhisk which he said had been used to transmit bolts of lightning to unsuspecting victims.

The 2,000-strong crowd began streaming to Msami on Friday morning from 27 surrounding villages. Word had gone out to all village headmen to bring their people for "smelling out." By mid-morning, all roads leading to Msami swarmed with men, women and children. They walked, rode in cars, lorries and carts pulled by oxen or donkeys. Among them were sick, old people who were said to have been given up by hospitals as hopeless cases.

All day on Friday and yesterday, the grounds of Msami looked like the venue for a mammoth political rally. Although ZANU (PF) is not officially involved and no directive was given from its 88 Manica Road headquarters in Salisbury to encourage him, Mr Chikanga works with ZANU (PF) officials in the area. He also carries two permits from the district commissioner and the local police.

A visiting ZANU (PF) political commissar "Comrade States," said he disapproved of what was going on. "I don't like it," he said. "The party must not be associated with it." Charges for the "sniffing out" are $1 a family and 50c for widows and old women.

Father Nigel Johnson, the Catholic head of St Paul's Mission, said: "I think that if this sort of thing is going to be encouraged, the liberation cause is lost. The people are paying $1 a family and they have to pay it. This man has already made thousands of dollars at Mrewa and Nyamutumbu. He is making more thousands here. These people have to come. Anyone who refuses to come is regarded as a witch. If the policy of the Government is *'pamberi nokubatana'* (forward with unity), this thing is destroying it. I would like to know where all this money is going, who is using it and who is exploiting the masses through fear. I also would like to know what's going to happen to people marked for life as witches when they go home—do they continue to live with their families?"

Amid cries of *"pasi nevaroyi"* (down with witches), Mr Chikanga started the proceedings by reading passages from the Bible referring to witchcraft. Then village headmen were called to stand in a row and their people lined up behind them.

The "smelling out" ceremony was a spine-chilling spectacle. The people looked frightened as—wild-eyed, shrieking like a devil and moving with a fast limp—Mr Chikanga romped among the lines wearing a crown of porcupine quills. His hand flashed in and out of the lines, touching those "smelt out." Frightened and shaken, they were dragged by chanting youths to the centre of the arena. Most of those dragged out were old men and women, grey haired and bent double with age.

It became even more bizarre when the alleged spirits, demons and witches began to grunt, roar, shriek and scream like wild animals. Mr Chikanga pointed out, however, that not all the people smelt out were witches. "Some are the suppressed spirits of *vadzimu* who would like to manifest themselves. Others are merely bad spirits which must be exorcised," he said.

He said he would give witches and people possessed by evil spirits certain medicines which would rid them of their evils. He said he would like the ZINATHA president, Dr Gordon Chavunduka, to assemble all the *ngangas* so that he could "smell out" the evil ones.

Sunday Mail, 21 June 1981

WITCH-HUNTS MUST STOP—MUZENDA

by Elton Mutasa

The Deputy Prime Minister, Mr Simon Muzenda, yesterday said the Government was concerned about developments in Mrewa and was considering taking action against a man involved in a witch-hunt in the district.

Addressing an Inter-District Conference of Mashonaland West in Hartley, Mr Muzenda told hundreds of delegates that the Government viewed the situation seriously and was considering taking appropriate action "to stop this nonsense in the area as quickly as possible."

The man at the centre of the storm, Mr Size Kapara Chikanga, held a ceremony in the district on Saturday where he "smelt out" more than 250 alleged witches, spirits (*vadzimu*) and evil forces (*mashave*) from among a crowd of about 3,000 people.

During his speech—interspersed with tremendous applause and ululation—the Deputy Prime Minister said those who caused terror and confusion among the people "cannot be tolerated in an independent Zimbabwe." The Deputy Prime Minister said there were many people who wanted only to swindle money from the people—a thing to which the Government "takes very serious exception. We are a people's Government working towards unity among all our people and we will not tolerate people who go around sowing seeds of disunity and hatred in Zimbabwe," he said.

No true *nganga* would go around telling people he could "smell out" witches and wizards and charge them money. Visibly angry, Mr

Muzenda said: "Such people are only bent on causing unnecessary havoc among our people—especially the tribesmen. He must be stopped. . . ." Speaking in Shona throughout, Mr Muzenda told his audience that there was no such thing as witchcraft and "our people must believe this."

He told delegates that Zimbabwe was not liberated to have its people terrorised by anybody. "What has happened in Mrewa is the highest form of intimidation which has to be stopped without delay. Right now that man could be holding Mrewa in his hands."

He also said ZANU (PF) would take action against its members who may go around "behaving like this under its name." He urged the delegates to end their meeting in a democratic manner and not to rush to a *nganga* to get *muti* [medicine] in order to be elected to higher positions. "People elect you because of what you are worth to them. If they know you are honest and work hard for them, then they will elect you."

He appealed to the people of Zimbabwe to stop slogans that abuse other political parties at this time "when we are trying to build a strong and united nation. Let's move forward together in unity irrespective of race, creed or tribe. We are Zimbabweans and we must build our country together."

Commenting on Saturday's witch-hunt in Mrewa, the president of the Zimbabwe National Traditional Healers Association, Professor Gordon Chavunduka, said that from his organisation's point of view, the job of a *nganga* was to cure people—nothing else.

ZINATHA was only concerned with trying to help sick people in society. The question of witchcraft, if it existed, was a matter for law and order and not medicine. Professor Chavunduka said he was not going to assemble his members as suggested by Mr Chikanga for a ceremony to "smell out" evil. "We are not going to undergo the test which Mr Chikanga suggests. We have a code of ethics in our organisation which all our members obey and there is no need for any other test. We are capable of disciplining any of our members who break the code of ethics and we are better qualified than Mr Chikanga who has avoided registering with us as other true *ngangas* have. Mr Chikanga must stop operating outside our medical framework," he said.

Herald, 22 June 1981

END THE HUNT

A report yesterday on the witch-hunting activities of a man in the Mrewa district made horrifying reading.

The mental and physical anguish suffered by the people who became his victims at a bizarre ceremony at Msami on Saturday must have been frightening in the extreme.

The whole sick affair must be halted, and quickly. What was even more astonishing about the report was a reference to the "legality" of the charade. The man is reported to be carrying permits from the district commissioner and the police.

To his credit a ZANU(PF) political commissar at the ceremony said that the party should not be associated with the witch-hunt. The Catholic head of St Paul's Mission, Father Nigel Johnson, rightly condemned the event.

And so, too, should all Zimbabweans. The Government must step in quickly to curb hysterical witch-hunting and other sinister practices associated with witches, spirits and evil forces.

Herald, 22 June 1981

MREWA "WITCH-HUNTER" IS BANNED

by Herald Reporters

The Government has banned a spirit medium, Mr Size Kapara Chikanga, from entering any of the former TTLs after reports that he was conducting massive "witch-hunts" in the Mrewa district.

Announcing the ban in an interview yesterday, the Minister of Local Government and Housing, Dr Edson Zvobgo, said that Mr Chikanga's activities were a "nuisance to public order and a threat to public peace." He condemned "collecting money through the practice of witch-hunting."

The *Sunday Mail* reported that Mr Chikanga held a ceremony near Mrewa at the weekend at which he "smelt-out" 250 alleged witches, spirits and evil forces among a crowd of 3,000.

Families were said to have been charged $1 for each "witch" uncovered and 50c for each "spirit" or "force." Mr Chikanga, it was said, claimed to have permission from the district administration for his activities. Police said yesterday they had started an investigation into the alleged witch-hunting, but sources said they had been hampered by the fact that Mr Chikanga was a registered member of the Zimbabwe National Traditional Healers' Association. ZINATHA's administrative secretary, Mr Taino Benhura, confirmed this yesterday, but said that Mr Chikanga faced expulsion if the "smelling-out" allegations were proved.

Mr Benhura said that Mr Size Chikanga should not be confused with Mr Brighton Chikanga, also practicing in the Mrewa district, whom he described as a "famous *nganga*" involved only in traditional healing.

Meanwhile, Mr Walter Patsanza, acting district commissioner for Mrewa, strongly denied Mr Size Chikanga's reported claim that he was operating under a permit issued by local officials. "It is not true," Mr Patsanza said. "I never issued him with such a permit, and I have established that none of my staff did."

Herald, 23 June 1981

APPENDIX 11

THE ZIMBABWEAN author, Dambudzo Marachera (1978), incorporated the *njuzu* as a symbol in his own myth making. *Njuzu* are said to have pale skins and fair hair like white people, and to live in villages beneath the water. They take selected people under the water, train them as healers, and return them to the living only if their kin do not cry for them but sacrifice an animal to the spirits at the water's edge. *Njuzu* are powerful spirits and much feared, although they grant healing powers. Like Henry James, Marachera dips into the "deep well of unconscious cerebration" and pours out a nightmare the ingredients of which are supplied from the "general vision of evil." The piece begins with an idyllic scene on a river bank. The author draws in danger (from father, kin, whites, spirits, animals, and water) to build to a crescendo of horror. The negative side of power is revealed (manfish, the *njuzu* that can heal or drown people or drive them mad in possessing them).

I had named the valley Lesapi after my birthplace where once I had learned to fish, to swim and to lie back into the soft green grass and relax, with my eyes closed and my head ringing with the cawing of the crows and the leisurely moo of cows grazing on My Robert's side of the river, where it was fenced and there was a notice about trespassers. And in the summer the white people held rubber-boat races on the river and sometimes I was allowed to watch them swirling along in the breezy hold of the river. But somebody drowned one day and my father told me not to go down to the river any more because the drowned boy would have turned into a manfish and he would want to have company in the depths of the waters. Water was good, but only when it did not have a manfish in it. My first nightmare was about a white manfish which materialised in my room and licked its great jaws at me and came towards my bed and said: "Come, come, come with me," and it raised its hand and drew a circle on the wall behind my head and said, "That circle will always bleed until you come to me." I looked at his hand and the fingers were webbed, with livid skin attaching each finger to another finger. And then he stretched out his index finger and touched my cheek with it. It was like being touched by a red-hot spike; and I cried out, but I could not hear my own voice: and they were trying to break down the door, and I cried out louder and the wooden door splintered apart and father rushed in with a world war in his eyes. But the manfish had gone; and there was a black frog squatting where he had been. The next day the medicine-man came and examined me and shook his head and said that an enemy had done it. He named Barbara's father, and my father bought strong medicine which would make what had been done to me boomerang on Barbara's father. They then made little incisions on my face and on my chest and rubbed a black powder into them, and said that should I ever come near water I must say to myself: "Help me, grandfather." My grandfather was dead, but they said that his spirit was always looking and watching over me. They made a fire and cast the black frog into it, and the medicine man said he would seed its ashes in Barbara's father's garden. But he could do nothing about the circle on the wall, because although I could clearly see it no one else could. Shortly after this, my eyes dimmed a little and I have had to wear spectacles since then; at the time, however, it only made the little circle jump sharply at me each time I entered my room. The spot where the manfish had touched me swelled with pus, and mother had to boil water with lots of salt and then squeeze the pus out and bathe it with the salted water; after that it healed a little, and ever since I have always had a little black mark there on my face. Soon afterwards Barbara's father went mad and one day his body was fished out of the river by police divers who wore black fish-suits. There were various abrasions on his face and the body was utterly naked, and something in the river seemed to have tried to eat him—there were curious tooth-marks on his buttocks and his shoulders had been partially eaten; the hands looked as though something had chewed them and tried to gnaw them from the arms.

APPENDIX 12

IT IS difficult to estimate how seriously accusations of witchcraft are taken. It seems to me that it often means little. To have the effects of witchcraft identified in a patient serves, frequently, as a warning to the family to put their house in order. Sometimes, however, accusations reverberate around the neighborhood and must be felt by the suspect if only in the way neighbors both avoid her and are carefully respectful toward her. Accusations (leveled by more than one person) against five people in Musami were brought to my attention, but there was never mention of steps that might be taken against them. It is against the law of the country even to name a witch (see Chavunduka 1982). I have on record over fifty cases in which witchcraft was said to have played a part in causing ill health or distress to someone. Children were carefully told which homes to avoid and they were instructed never to eat food prepared at those homesteads.

APPENDIX 13

FOUR *N'ANGA* identified the 11 plants used in Test A: the uses to which they put the plants fall within those given in Gelfand et al. (1985) and Wild (1972).

1. Shona name: Scientific name:
   mudima   *Dalbergia nitidula*
   (Wild, 13)

Tree. In Gelfand et al. (145).

2. Shona name: Scientific name:
   murungu   *Ozoroa insignus*
   (Wild, 54)   subspecies *reticulata*

Shrub or small tree. Gelfand et al. (172–73).

3. Shona name: Scientific name:
   mupfeyo   *Xerophyta equisetoides*
   (Wild, 49)

Gelfand et al. (109).

4. Shona name: Scientific name:
   musvisvinwa   *Fadogia ancylantha*
   (Gelfand et al., 323).

Makoni tea. Gelfand et al. (224).

5. Shona name: Scientific name:
   mukuc/ciyo   *Pseudolachnastylis maprouneifolia*

Deciduous tree. Gelfand et al. (167).

6. Shona name: Scientific name:
    musikavakadzi   *Vernonia amygdalina*
    (Wild, 59)

Erect subshrub. Wild says that the Shona name literally means "creates women" and the plant is used to help women conceive daughters and for gynecological problems. Gelfand et al. (238-39).

7. Shona name: Scientific name:
    muroro   *Annona senegalensis*
    (Wild, 54)

Wild custard apple. Gelfand et al. (125-26).

8. Shona name: Scientific name:
    muwore   *Adenia gummifera*
    (Wild, 75)

Monkey rope—a woody-tendriled climber. Gelfand et al. (190).

9. Shona name: Scientific name:
    zheverashuro   *Inula glomerata*
    (Gelfand et al., 333)

Hare's ear. Gelfand et al. (235-36).

10. Shona name: Scientific name:
    mufufu   *Securidaca longipedunculata*
    (Wild, 17)

Shrub or small tree. Gelfand et al. (160-62).

11. Shona name: Scientific name:
    bepu   *Combretum platypetalum*
    (Wild, 4)

Subshrub with annual stems from a woody root-crown. Gelfand et al. (194-95).

APPENDIX 14

HANNAN (1984) gives the following definitions:

n'anga Diviner-healer. Dealer in medicines and charms.
chiremba 1. Doctor. 2. Healer (title with which *n'anga* is addressed). 3.
Hospital orderly.
svikiro Medium (generally of tribal spirit).

Gelfand understood that *nganga* (*n'anga*) either divine or heal:

> There are two main types of practitioners among the *nganga*,
> diviners and herbalists. Distinguishing them according to their
> functions, one could say that the young *nganga* has a choice of
> specialising either as a diagnostician or as a therapeutist. The
> diviner, through the medium of his *shave,* finds out which spirit
> is responsible for the illness, usually communicating with his
> spirit through his *hakata* or divining bones. The herbalist, on
> the other hand, is not concerned with the cause of illness, but
> only with the treatment of physical symptoms. But he also relies
> on his *shave* to show him where to find the appropriate herbs,
> the information being supplied to him in dreams. There are,
> however, some *nganga* who are able to divine as well as treat
> with herbs. [1964, 63]

Gelfand et al. described three types of traditional healers: "N'anga
who divine with the aid of their healing spirits without *hakata* are by
far the largest group, and are followed by those who use divining de-
vices. The smallest group is composed of *n'anga* who provide medicines only and do not divine" (1985, 22).

ZINATHA, as reported in the *Herald,* 20 April 1982, defines healers
in this way:

N'ANGAS NOW MEN OF LETTERS

All spirit mediums and general traditional practitioners are required to indicate their qualifications after their names, says the president of Zimbabwe National Traditional Healers Association (ZINATHA), Professor Gordon Chavunduka.

Spirit mediums must write the letters SM after their names and traditional practitioners must have TMP after theirs. Those who practise as both must indicate so by including the two abbreviations.

This was to comply with the Traditional Medical Practitioners Act No. 38 of 1981, said Dr. Chavunduka in a statement. He added that traditional healers were of three main types: Spirit mediums who only carry out diagnosis but do not handle medicines. General traditional healers who used to be called herbalists. Those who are spirit mediums but also treat patients.

Among the sixty healers with whom I worked only one (apart from the men who sold *materia medica* in the urban marketplaces) said he was only a herbalist and not a diviner. All the others both divined and treated patients.

APPENDIX 15

THE FOLLOWING report is from the *Sunday Mail*, 30 January 1983:

WITCH-HUNTING

That witch-hunting is still being practised in this day and age, splitting families and imposing torture on innocent people so accused is both scandalous and incongruous.

Witch-hunting is based on the absurd and unscientific belief that all deaths, be they suicides, car accidents, what have you or whether they are the deaths of people who are 200 years old, are caused by human beings called witches.

A related crying absurdity is the childish belief that only Africans can be bewitched; other races cannot be bewitched.

When ZINATHA was formed, it was thought that it would cleanse traditional medicine of the primitive and satanic aspect of witchcraft promotion and belief.

But what is discernible is that, instead, it is giving respectability to witchcraft beliefs and to the *n'angas* who are not willing to give up witch-hunting because if they do so they lose more than half their income.

Professor Gordon Chavunduka, despite what he says in defence of ZINATHA *n'angas,* must admit that they are spreading a superstitious and dangerous belief in witchcraft, using him and the association as a shield.

As long as this mentally stultifying, superstitious belief retains a hold on the people, there can be no progress in our country, let alone development along the scientific socialist path.

ZINATHA is the "blue surf" of *n'angas* who are dedicated to the development of backwardness in Zimbabwe by promoting the superstitious belief in non-existent witchcraft.

This is not surprising when it is remembered that *n'angaism* is the only profession that is not learnt, but is merely dreamt and claimed.

The following is an excerpt from the *Herald,* 8 December 1989, p. 20:

ZIFA MAKE HISTORY AS THE NATIONAL TEAM,
CLUB SIDES FAIL TO IMPRESS

The 1989 soccer season ended, as so many have in the last few years, with the survival and success of the fittest on the domestic scene and the continuing worries over our national team's performances in the African Nations Cup and World Cup competitions. Senior sportswriter Sam Marisa looks back on another traumatic year when the Dynamos double, ground shutouts and "juju's" remarkable appeal all made people sit up and take notice.

On a sad note though there were a number of incidents that gave our soccer adverse publicity.

There was an upsurge on the number of superstition related incidents with some clubs seen urinating in front of spectators "as per doctors prescription" in order to win.

One of the most talked about incidents occurred a few hours before the kick off of the Zifa Cup final between Dynamos and Highlanders at the National Sports Stadium.

Prior to the start of the match, Dynamos officials apprehended a groundsman who they accused of being a Highlanders agent sent to put "muti" on the pitch.

In a bid to avoid being bewitched, Dynamos refused to use designated entry points. The matter has been brought before the disciplinary committee.

No decision has been passed by the disciplinary committee and observers are convinced that no action will be taken as the two clubs are believed to be more powerful than the association.

Surprisingly Zifa handed out life sentences on soft targets—Tongogara—which were later rescinded.

APPENDIX 16

THE FOLLOWING extract is from Ziana, the *Herald,* 8 March 1989:

TWO TO HANG FOR MURDERING 15-YEAR-OLD

Two men who were part of a group of five who killed a 15-year-old boy and cut out his heart for purposes of appeasing an evil spirit were sentenced to death by the High Court in Harare recently. . . .

The body of the deceased was found mutilated on August 27, 1988.

The court heard that the group, which included the deceased's father, strangled the boy who was coming back home from his aunt's home and removed his heart in order to satisfy a belief in witchcraft.

Evidence was that Masimba's sister was possessed by an evil spirit. Her father . . . consulted a traditional healer . . . who advised him that the problem would only be solved by offering a human heart. A traditional ceremony was then held . . . in July where it was agreed that a child be killed and the heart be removed to appease the evil spirit.

Five men, including the deceased's father, were alleged to have agreed that Masimba was the child to be killed and that according to their plan, Masimba should be sent by his father to his aunt's home, Maude, who was married to the traditional healer, Ali, to discuss the sale of a donkey.

The next day on July 29, after he had been given $85 by Ali, Masimba left for home.

Maude alleged that soon after Masimba left her home, he was in the company of her husband Ali and Sibanda.

In his defence outline, Ali admitted he was consulted in his capacity as a traditional healer by the deceased's father, whom he advised that the evil spirit could only be appeased by sacrificing a beast, and denied taking part in the actual killing of the boy.

He claimed Sibanda and another man, Josias, held the deceased at the request of his father who actually strangled the boy.

Sibanda, who denied participating in the killing of the boy, alleged Ali grabbed the deceased while his father strangled him.

The State was represented by Mr John Small, of the Attorney General's Office.

Ali was represented by Mr Erick Mhlanga and Sibanda by Mr Arthur Manase.

BIBLIOGRAPHY

ANPPCAN (African Network on Prevention and Protection against Child Abuse and Neglect). 1987. "Children in Situations of Armed Conflict in Africa." Selected papers from the Conference on Children in Situations of Armed Conflict in Africa: An Agenda for Action, 6–10 July, Nairobi.

Aries, P. 1962. *Centuries of Childhood.* London: Jonathan Cape.

Asad, T. 1986. "The Concept of Cultural Translation in British Social Anthropology." In *Writing Culture: Twentieth-Century Ethnography, Literature and Art,* edited by J. Clifford and G. Marcus. Cambridge: Harvard University Press.

Aschwanden, H. 1987. *Symbols of Death: An Analysis of the Consciousness of the Karanga.* Gweru: Mambo Press.

Bachelard, G. 1971. *The Poetics of Reverie, Childhood, Language and the Cosmos.* Translated by D. Russell. Boston: Beacon Press.

Beach, D. N. 1980. *The Shona and Zimbabwe, 900–1850.* Gwelo: Mambo Press.

Bellow, S. 1989. *The Bellarosa Connection.* Harmondsworth: Penguin.

Benatar, S. R. 1986. "Ethical and Moral Issues in Contemporary Medical Practice." Proceedings of an 'in-house' conference, Faculty of Medicine, University of Cape Town, 7–8 August 1985.

Berglund, A. 1976. *Zulu Thought-Patterns and Symbolism.* London: Hurst.

————. 1989. "Confessions of Guilt and Restorations to Health: Some Illustrative Zulu Examples." In *Culture, Experience and Pluralism: Essays on African Ideas of Illness and Healing,* edited by A. Jacobson Widding and D. Westerlund. Uppsala: Almquist and Wiksell International.

Bernardi, B. 1950. "The Social Structure of the Kraal among the Zezuru in Musami, Southern Rhodesia." In *Communications from the School of African Studies* (23). Cape Town: University of Cape Town.

Bloch, M., and J. Parry, eds. 1982. *Death and the Regeneration of Life.* Cambridge: Cambridge University Press.

Bourdieu, P. 1977. *Outline of a Theory in Practice.* Translated by R. Nice. Cambridge: Cambridge University Press.

———. 1990. *In Other Words. Essays Towards a Reflexive Sociology.* Cambridge: Polity Press.

Bourdillon, M. F. C. 1981. "Suggestions of Bureaucracy in Korekore Religion: Putting the Ethnography Straight." *Zambezia* 9(2): 119–36.

———. 1982. "Freedom and Constraint among Shona Spirit Mediums." In *Religious Organization and Religious Experience,* edited by J. Davis. London: Academic Press.

———. 1983. "Religious Symbols and Political Change." Seminar paper, Department of Sociology, University of Zimbabwe.

———. 1984–85. "Religious Symbols and Political Change." *Zambezia* 12:39–54.

———. 1987a. "Guns and Rain: Taking Structural Analysis Too Far?" Review Article. *Africa* 57(2): 263–74.

———. 1987b. *The Shona Peoples. An Ethnography of the Contemporary Shona, with special reference to their Religion.* Gweru: Mambo Press. First published 1976.

Bourdillon, M. F. C., and P. Gundani. 1988. "Rural Christians and the Zimbabwe Liberation War: A Case Study." In *Christianity South of the Zambezi.* Vol. 3, *Church and State in Zimbabwe,* edited by C. F. Hallencreutz and A. Moyo. Gweru: Mambo Press.

Browman, D. C., and R. A. Schwarz, eds. 1979. *Spirits, Shamans, and Stars: Perspectives from South America.* The Hague: Mouton.

Bullock, C. 1927. *The Mashona (The Indigenous Natives of S. Rhodesia).* Cape Town: Juta.

Bundy, C. 1993. "At War with the Future? Black South African Youth in the 1990s" In *South Africa: The Political Economoy of Transformation,* edited by S. Stedman. Boulder, Colorado: Lynn Riemer.

Carothers, J. C. 1970. *The African Mind in Health and Disease: A Study in Ethnopsychiatry.* New York: Negro Universities Press. First published in 1953.

Carrithers, M., S. Collins, and S. Les, eds. 1985. *The Category of the Person: Anthropology, Philosophy, History.* Cambridge: Cambridge University Press.

CCJP (Catholic Commission for Justice and Peace in Rhodesia). 1977. "Rhodesia: The Propaganda War." Salisbury: Catholic Commission for Justice and Peace.

Centre of African Studies, University of Edinburgh. 1986. "African Medicine in the Modern World." Seminar Proceedings, no. 27 (10-11 December). Edinburgh: Centre of African Studies.

Chavunduka, G. L. 1970. "Social Change in a Shona Ward." Occasional Paper no. 4, Department of Sociology, University of Rhodesia.

———. 1978. *Traditional Healers and the Shona Patient.* Gwelo: Mambo Press.

———. 1982. "Witches, Witchcraft and the Law in Zimbabwe." ZINATHA Occasional Paper no. 1, Harare.

Cheater, A. P. 1981. "Effects of the Liberation War in One Commercial Farming Area of Zimbabwe." Seminar paper, Department of Sociology, University of Zimbabwe. Mimeograph.

Cilliers, J. K. 1985. *Counter-Insurgency in Rhodesia.* Dover, N.H.: Croom Helm.

Clifford, J. 1986. "Introduction." In *Writing Culture: The Poetics and Politics of Ethnography.* Berkelely: University of California Press.

———. 1988. *The Predicament of Culture: Twentieth-Century Ethnography, Literature and Art.* Cambridge: Harvard University Press.

———. 1992. "Traveling Cultures." In *Cultural Studies,* edited by L. Grossberg, C. Nelson, and P. R. Treichler. New York: Routledge.

Clifford, J., and G. Marcus, eds. 1986. *Writing Culture: The Poetics and Politics of Ethnography.* Berkeley: University of California Press.

Crapanzano, V. 1973. *The Hamadsha. A Study in Moroccan Ethnopsychiatry.* Berkeley: University of California Press.

———. 1980. *Tuhami. Portrait of a Moroccan.* Chicago: University of Chicago Press.

Crawford, J. R. 1967. *Witchcraft and Sorcery in Rhodesia.* London: Oxford University Press.

Cunningham, A. B. 1988. "Investigation of the Herbal Medicine Trade in Natal/Kwazulu." Investigational Report no. 29, Institute of National Resources, University of Natal.

Dawes, A., and D. Donald. 1994. *Childhood and Adversity: Psychological Perspectives from South African Research.* Cape Town: David Philip.

Demos, J. P. 1982. *Entertaining Satan: Witchcraft and the Culture of Early New England.* New York: Oxford University Press.

Devisch, R. 1985. "Perspectives of Pluralism: An Ethnographic Approach." In *Theoretical Explorations in African Religion,* edited by W. Van Binsbergen and M. Schoffeleers. London: Routledge and Kegan Paul.

Dodge, C. P., and M. Raundalen, eds. 1987. *War, Violence and Children in Uganda.* Oslo: Norwegian University Press.

Draft Convention on the Rights of the Child, The. 1988. International Children's Rights Monitor 5(1), supplement.

Drummond, R. B., M. Gelfand, and S. Mavi. 1975. "Medicinal and Other Uses of Succulents by the Rhodesian African." *Excelsa* 5:51–56.

Edel, L., ed. 1971. *Henry James: Stories of the Supernatural.* London: Barrie and Jenkins.

Eribon, D. 1991. *Michel Foucault.* Cambridge: Harvard Universitry Press.

Erikson, E. H. 1950. *Childhood and Society.* 2d ed. New York: W. W. Norton.

Erny, P. 1973. *Childhood and the Cosmos: The Social Psychology of the Black African Child.* Translated by A. Mboukou. Washington, D.C.: Black Orpheus Press. First published in French, 1968.

Evans-Pritchard, E. E. 1937. *Witchcraft, Oracles, and Magic among the Azande.* Oxford: Clarendon Press.

————. 1965. *Theories of Primitive Religion.* Oxford: Clarendon Press.

————. 1981. *A History of Anthropological Thought.* London: Faber and Faber.

————. 1982. "Witchcraft amongst the Azande." In *Witchcraft and Sorcery,* edited by M. Marwick. Harmondsworth, Middlesex: Penguin. First published in 1929.

Fabian, J. 1985. "Religious Pluralism: An Ethnographic Approach." In *Theoretical Explorations African Religion,* edited by W. Van Binsbergen and M. Schoffeleers. London: Routledge and Kegan Paul.

Favret-Saada, J. 1980. *Deadly Words: Witchcraft in the Bocage.* Translated by C. Cullen. Cambridge: Cambridge University Press. First published in French, 1977.

Feierman, S. 1979. *Health and Society in Africa: A Working Bibliography.* Waltham: African Studies Association.

―――. 1984. "The Social Origins of Health and Healing in Africa." Paper commissioned by the ACLS/SSRC Joint Committee on African Studies for presentation at the 27th annual meeting of the African Studies Association. 25–28 October, Los Angeles.

Feyerabend, P. 1978. *Against Method Outline of an Anarchistic Theory of Knowledge.* London: Verso.

Firth, R. 1973. *Symbols, Public and Private.* London: George Allen and Unwin.

Fortes, M. 1987. *Religion, Morality and the Person: Essays on Tallensi Religion.* Edited and with an introduction by Jack Goody. Cambridge: Cambridge University Press.

Foster, G. M., and B. G. Anderson. 1978. *Medical Anthropology.* New York: Wiley.

Foucault, M. 1973. *The Order of Things: An Archaeology of the Human Sciences.* New York: Vintage Books.

―――. 1984. *The Foucault Reader.* Edited by P. Rabinow. New York: Pantheon Books.

―――. 1987. *Mental Illness and Psychology,* translated by A. Sheridan. Berkeley: University of California Press. First published in French, 1954.

―――. 1988. *Technologies of the Self: A Seminar with Michel Foucault.* Edited by L. H. Martin, H. Gutman, and P. H. Hutton. London: Tavistock.

Frederikse, J. 1982. *None But Ourselves: Masses vs. Media in the Making of Zimbabwe.* Johannesburg: Ravan Press.

Freud, A. 1981. *Psychoanalytic Psychology of Normal Development, 1970–1980.* London: Hogarth Press.

Fry, P. 1976. *Spirits of Protest: Spirit-Mediums and the Articulation of Consensus among the Zezuru of Southern Rhodesia (Zimbabwe).* Cambridge: Cambridge University Press.

Fyfe, C. 1986. "African Medicine in the Modern World." Proceedings of a seminar held in the Centre of African Studies, University of Edinburgh.

Garbett, G. K. 1960. "Growth and Change in a Shona Ward." Occasional Paper no. 1, Department of African Studies, University College of Rhodesia and Nyasaland.

————. 1987. "Symbolic Labour and the Transfer of Symbolic Capital in the Production of a Ritual Field among Korekore and Zezuru of Zimbabwe." *Social Analysis* 22:47–60.

Geertz, C. 1988. *Works and Lives: The Anthropologist as Author.* Cambridge: Polity Press.

Gelfand, M. 1956. *Medicine and Magic of the Mashona.* Cape Town: Juta.

————. 1959. *Shona Ritual.* Cape Town: Juta.

————. 1964. *Witch Doctor: Traditional Medicine Man of Rhodesia.* London: Havill Press.

————. 1967. *The African Witch, with Particular Reference to Witchcraft Beliefs Practised among the Shona of Rhodesia.* Edinburgh: Livingstone.

————. 1977. *The Spiritual Beliefs of the Shona: A Case Study Based on Field Work among the East-Central Shona.* Gwelo: Mambo Press.

————. 1979. *Growing Up in Shona Society.* Gwelo: Mambo Press.

————. 1982. "The Traditional Shona Diet." *Zimbabwe Science News* 16(6), 10–24.

Gelfand, M., S. Mavi, and R. B. Drummond. 1977. "An Account of the Treatment of a Psychiatric Patient by a *N'anga.*" *Central African Journal of Medicine* 23(7), 158–61.

Gelfand, M., S. Mavi, R. B. Drummond, and B. Ndemera. 1985. *The Traditional Medical Practitioner in Zimbabwe: His Principles of Practice and Pharmacopoeia.* Gweru: Mambo Press.

Gelfand, M., S. Mavi, and R. Loewenson. 1981. " The Urban *N'anga* in Practice." *Central African Journal of Medicine* 27(5): 93–95.

Giddens, A. 1979. *Central Problems in Social Theory, Action, Structure and Contradiction in Social Analysis.* London: Macmillan.

————. 1984. *The Constitution of Society: Outline of the Theory of Structuration.* Cambridge: Polity Press.

Gluck, S. B., and D. Patai, eds. 1991. *Women's Words: The Feminist Practice of Oral History.* New York: Routledge.

Gluckman, H. M. 1936. "The Realm of the Supernatural among the South-Eastern Bantu." Doctoral dissertation, Oxford University.

————. 1963. *Custom and Conflict in Africa.* Oxford: Basil Blackwell.

Gordon, L. 1984. "A Writer's Life." In *Virginia Woolf: A Centenary Perspective,* edited by Eric Warner. London: Macmillan.

Hamutyinei, M. A., and A.B. Plangger. 1987. *Tsumo-Shumo. Shona Proverbial Lore and Wisdom*. 2d ed., rev. Gweru: Mambo Press.

Hannan, M. 1959. *Standard Shona Dictionary*. 2d ed. Salisbury: Mardon Printers.

———. 1984. *Standard Shona Dictionary*. Rev. ed. with addendum. Harare: College Press.

Harris, G. G. 1978. *Casting Out Anger: Religion among the Taita of Kenya*. Cambridge: Cambridge University Press.

Heald, S. 1989. *Controlling Anger: The Sociology of Gisu Violence*. Manchester: Manchester University Press.

Heelas, P., and A. Lock, eds. 1981. *Indigenous Psychologies: The Anthropology of Self*. London: Academic Press.

Heilbroner, R. L. 1980. *Marxism: For and Against*. New York: W. W. Norton.

Heilbrun, C. G. 1989. *Writing a Woman's Life*. London: Women's Press.

Heller, E. 1988. *The Importance of Nietzsche: Ten Essays*. Chicago: University of Chicago Press.

Hove, M. M. 1985. *Confessions of a Wizard*. Gweru: Mambo Press.

Hutton, P. H. 1988. "Foucault, Freud, and the Technologies of the Self." In *Technologies of the Self: A Seminar with Michel Foucault*, edited by L. H. Martin, H. Gutman, and P. H. Hutton. London: Tavistock.

Jacobson-Widding, A., and D. Westerlund, eds. 1989. *Culture, Experience and Pluralism: Essays on African Ideas of Illness and Healing*. Uppsala: Acta Universitatis Upsaliensis.

James, H. 1971. "The Turn of the Screw." In *Henry James. Stories of the Supernatural*, edited by L. Edel. London: Barrie and Jenkins. First published in 1898.

Janzen, J. M. 1978. *The Quest for Therapy: Medical Pluralism in Lower Zaire*. Berkeley: University of California Press.

———. 1982. *Lemba, 1650–1930. A Drum of Affliction in Africa and the New World*. New York: Garland.

———. 1985. "The Consequences of Literacy in African Religion: The Kongo Case." In *Lemba, 1650–1930. A Drum of Affliction in Africa and the New World* by J. M. Janzen. New York: Garland.

Jedrej, M. C., and R. Shaw, eds. 1992. *Dreaming, Religion and Society in Africa*. Leiden: E. J. Brill

Joyce, J. 1957. *Finnegan's Wake*. New York: Viking.

Jung, C. G. 1954. "The Development of Personality." In *Collected Works*, vol. 17. London: Routledge Kegan Paul.

―――. 1968. *Analytical Psychology: Its Theory and Practice: The Tavistock Lectures*. London: Routledge and Kegan Paul.

Kidd, D. 1969. *Savage Childhood: A Study of Kafir Children*. New York: Negro Universities Press. First published in 1906.

Kiernan, J. P. 1982. "The 'Problem of Evil' in the Context of Ancestral Intervention in the Affairs of the Living in Africa." *Man* 17: 287-301.

Kleinman, A. 1980. *Patients and Healers in the Context of Culture: An Exploration of the Borderland between Anthropology, Medicine, and Psychiatry*. Berkeley: University of California Press.

―――. 1986. *Social Origins of Distress and Disease: Depression, Neurasthenia, and Pain in Modern China*. New Haven: Yale University Press.

Krige, J. D. 1982. "The Social Function of Witchcraft." In *Witchcraft and Sorcery*, edited by M. Marwick. Harmondsworth, Middlesex: Penguin. First published in 1947.

Krige, N. 1988. "The Zimbabwean War of Liberation: Struggles within the Struggle." *Journal of Southern African Studies* 14(2): 304-22.

Kuper, A. 1983. "The Structure of Dream Sequences." In *Culture, Medicine and Psychiatry* 7:153-75.

La Fontaine, J. S. 1985a. *Initiation: Ritual Drama and Secret Knowledge across the World*. Harmondsworth: Penguin.

―――. 1985b. "Person and Individual: Some Anthropological Reflections." In *The Category of the Person. Anthropology, Philosophy, History*, edited by M. Carrithers, S. Collins, and S. Lukes. Cambridge: Cambridge University Press.

Lan, D. 1984. "Spirit Mediums and the Authority to Resist in the Struggle for Zimbabwe." In *The Societies of Southern Africa in the 19th and 20th Centuries*, vol. 13. Collected Seminar Papers, no. 33: 152-61. London: Institute of Commonwealth Studies, University of London.

―――. 1985. *Guns and Rain: Guerrillas and Spirit Mediums in Zimbabwe*. London: James Currey.

Last, M. 1979. "Strategies against Time." *Sociology of Health and Illness* 1(13): 306-17.

_____. 1981. "The Importance of Knowing About Not Knowing." *Social Science of Medicine* 15B(3): 387–92.

Last, M., and G. L. Chavunduka, eds. 1986. *The Professionalisation of African Medicine*. Manchester: Manchester University Press in association with the International African Institute.

Laubscher, B. J. F. 1937. *Sex, Custom and Psychopathology: A Study of South African Pagan Natives*. London: George Routledge and Sons.

Leach, E. 1982. *Social Anthropology*. Glasgow: Fontana Paperbacks.

Levy, R. I. 1973. *Tahitians: Mind and Experience in the Society Islands*. Chicago: University of Chicago Press.

Lewis, G. 1986. "The Look of Magic." *Man* 21(3), 414–37.

_____. 1993. "Double Standards of Treatment Evaluation." In *Knowledge, Power, and Practice: The Anthropology of Medicine and Everyday Life,* edited by S. Lindenbaum and M. Lock. Berkeley: University of California Press.

Lewis, I. M. 1971. *Ecstatic Religion: An Anthropological Study of Spirit Possession and Shamanism*. Harmondsworth: Penguin.

_____, ed. 1977. *Symbols and Sentiments: Cross-Cultural Studies in Symbolism*. London: Academic Press.

Lienhardt, G. 1985. "Self: Public, Private: Some African Representations." In *The Category of the Person: Anthropology, Philosophy, History,* edited by M. Carrithers, S. Collins, and S. Lukes. Cambridge; Cambridge University Press.

Lindenbaum, S., and M. Lock., eds. 1993. *Knowledge, Power, and Practice: The Anthropology of Medicine and Everyday Life*. Berkeley: University of California Press.

Macfarlane, A. 1985. "The Root of All Evil." In *The Anthropology of Evil,* edited by D. Parkin. Oxford: Basil Blackwell.

MacGaffey, W. 1972. "Comparative Analysis of Central African Religions." *Africa* 42:21–31.

Mafico, T. J., and G. L. Chavunduka. 1986. "Witchcraft: Belief and Realities: A Debate." *Zambezia* 13(2): 119–37.

Mannheim, K. 1927. *Essays in the Sociology of Knowledge*. London: Routledge and Kegan Paul.

Marachera, D. 1978. *House of Hunger: Short Stories*. Harare: Zimbabwe Publishing House.

Marwick, M., ed. 1982. *Witchcraft and Sorcery. Selected Readings*. Harmondsworth: Penguin. First published in 1970.

Marx, K. 1968. "Theses on Feuerbach." In *Selected Works,* by K. Marx and F. Engels. Moscow: Progress.

Matteson-Langdon, E. J., and G. Baer, eds. 1992. *Portals of Power: Shamanism in South America.* Albuquerque: University of New Mexico Press.

Mauss, M. 1985. "A Category of the Human Mind: The Notion of Person; the Notion of Self." In *The Category of the Person: Anthropology, Philosophy, History,* edited by M. Carrithers, S. Collins, and S. Lukes. Cambridge: Cambridge University Press. First published in 1938.

Mayer, P. 1954. "Witches." Inaugural lecture delivered at Rhodes University, Grahamstown.

McClain, C. S., ed. 1989. *Women as Healers: Cross-Cultural Perspectives.* New Brunswick, N.J.: Rutgers University Press.

McNay, L. 1992. *Foucault and Feminism: Power, Gender and the Self.* Cambridge: Polity Press.

Middleton, J., and E. H. Winter, eds. 1963. *Witchcraft and Sorcery in East Africa.* London: Routledge and Kegan Paul.

Midgley, M. 1986. *Wickedness. A Philosophical Essay.* London: Ark Paperbacks. First published in 1984.

Moore-King, B. 1988. *White Man, Black War.* Harare: Baobab Books.

Moyo, J. Z., Social History Project. Forthcoming. *So That Our Youngsters Will Know.* Harare: Baobab Books.

Needham, R. 1981. "Inner States as Universals: Sceptical Reflections on Human Nature." In *Indigenous Psychologies: The Anthropology of Self,* edited by P. Heelas and A. Lock. London: Academic Press.

Ngubane, H. 1977. *Body and Mind in Zulu Medicine: An Ethnography of Health and Disease in Nyuswa-Zulu Thought and Practice.* London: Academic Press.

Nyazema, N. Z. 1984a. "Crocodile Bile, A Poison: Myth or Reality?" *Central African Journal of Medicine* 30(6): 102–3.

———. 1984b. "Poisoning due to Traditional Remedies." *Central African Journal of Medicine* 30(5): 80–83.

Olupona, J. K., ed. 1991. *African Traditional Religions in Contemporary Society.* New York: Paragon House.

Overing, J., ed. 1985a. *Reason and Morality.* London: Tavistock.

————. 1985b. "There is No End of Evil: The Guilty Innocents and their Fallible God." In *The Anthropology of Evil*, edited by D. Parkin. Oxford: Basil Blackwell.

————. n.d. "Personal Autonomy and the Domestication of the Self in Piaroa Society." In *Acquiring Culture: Cross Cultural Studies in Child Development*, edited by G. Jahoda and I. M. Lewis. London: Croom Helm.

Parkin, D., ed. 1985. *The Anthropology of Evil*. Oxford: Basil Blackwell.

Peek, P. M. 1991. *African Divination Systems: Ways of Knowing*. Bloomington: Indiana University Press.

Pierce, T. O. 1993. "Lay Medical Knowledge in an African Context." In *Knowledge, Power, and Practice: The Anthropology of Medicine in Everyday Life*. Berkeley: University of California Press.

Pocock, D. 1985. "Unruly Evil." In *The Anthropology of Evil*, edited by D. Parkin. Oxford: Basil Blackwell.

Pongweni, A. J. C. 1982. *Songs That Won the Liberation War*. Harare: College Press.

Popper, K. 1976. *Unended Quest. An Intellectual Autobiography*. Glasgow: Fontana. First published in 1974.

Posselt, F. W. T. 1935. *Fact and Fiction. A Short Account of the Natives of Southern Rhodesia*. Bulawayo: Rhodesian Printing and Publishing Company.

Progress Reports on Health and Development in Southern Africa. 1989 (Fall/Winter). Washington, D.C.: Henry J. Kaiser Family Foundation.

Ranger, T. 1982. "The Death of Chaminuka: Spirit Mediums, Nationalism and the Guerilla War in Zimbabwe." *African Affairs* 18(324): 349–69.

————. 1985. *Peasant Consciousness and Guerrilla War in Zimbabwe*. A Comparative Study. Harare: Zimbabwe Publishing House.

Reynolds, P. 1986. "Concepts of Childhood Drawn from the Ideas and Practice of Traditional Healers in Musami." *Zambezia* 13(1): 1–10.

————. 1986. "The Training of Traditional Healers in Mashonaland" in Murray Last and G. L. Chavunduka (eds.) *The Professionalisation of African Medicine*. Manchester: Manchester University Press in association with the International African Institute.

Rorty, R. 1986 "The Contingency of Selfhood." Northcliffe Lecture, University College, London.

Schoffeleers, J. M. 1978. *Guardians of the Land: Essays on Central African Territorial Cults.* Gwelo: Mambo Press.

———. 1987. "Peasants, Mediums and Guerillas." Review article. *Journal of Southern African Studies* 14(1): 147–52.

Scott, J. C. 1985. *Weapons of the Weak: Everyday Forms of Peasant Resistance.* New Haven: Yale University Press.

Selous, F. C. 1981. *A Hunter's Wanderings in Africa.* Bulawayo: Books of Zimbabwe. Facsimile reprint of the 1881 edition.

———. 1983. *Travel and Adventure in South-East Africa.* London: R. Ward. Facsimile reprint of the 1883 edition.

Shone, D. K., and R. B. Drummond. 1965. "Poisonous Plants of Rhodesia." *Rhodesian Agricultural Journal* 62, (4): 1–64.

Singer, J. 1981. *Daydreaming and Fantasy.* Oxford: Oxford University Press.

Smartt, C. G. F. 1964. "Short-Term Treatment of the African Psychotic." *Central African Journal of Medicine* 10(9): 1–2.

Spencer, J. 1989. "Anthropology as a Kind of Writing." *Man* 24(1): 145–64.

Stewart, C. 1991. *Demons and the Devil.* Princeton: Princeton University Press.

Stott, R. et al. 1988. "Is Cooperation between Traditional and Western Healers Possible?" *Complementary Medical Research* 3(1): 15–22.

Swartz, L., and A. Levett. 1989. "Political Repression and Children in South Africa: The Social Construction of Damaging Effects." *Social Science and Medicine,* 28(7): 741–50.

———. 1990. "Political Oppression and Children in South Africa." In *Political Violence and the Struggle in South Africa,* edited by N. C. Manganyi and A. du Toit. London: Macmillan

Taussig, M. 1987. *Shamanism, Colonialism, and the Wild Man: A Study in Terror and Healing.* Chicago: University of Chicago Press.

Tedlock, B., ed. 1987. *Dreaming: Anthropological and Psychological Interpretations.* Cambridge: Cambridge University Press.

Turner, P. R. 1970. "Witchcraft as Negative Charisma." *Ethnology* 9:366–72.

Turner, V. 1961. "Ritual Symbolism, Morality and Social Structure among the Ndembu." *The Rhodes-Livingstone Journal, Human*

Problems in British Central Africa 30.

———. 1967. *The Forest of Symbols: Aspects of Ndembu ritual.* Ithaca, N.Y.: Cornell University Press.

———. 1981. *The Drums of Affliction: A Study of Religious Processes among the Ndembu of Zambia.* London: Hutchinson University Library for Africa. First published in 1968.

———. 1992. *Blazing the Trail: Way Marks in the Exploration of Symbols.* Tucson: University of Arizona Press.

Turton, R. W., G. Straker, and F. Moosa. 1991. "Experiences of Violence in the Lives of Township Youths in 'Unrest' and 'Normal' Conditions." *South African Journal of Psychology* 21(2): 55–77.

Tyler, S. A. 1987. *The Unspeakable. Discourse, Dialogue, and Rhetoric in the Postmodern World.* Madison: University of Wisconsin Press.

UNICEF 1989a. *Children on the Front Line: The Impact of Apartheid, Destabilization and Warfare on Children in Southern and South Africa.* 3d ed. New York: UNICEF.

———. 1989b. *The State of the World's Children 1989.* Oxford: Oxford University Press.

van Binsbergen, W., and M. Schoffeleers, eds. 1985. *Theoretical Explorations in African Religion.* London: Routledge and Kegan Paul.

Werbner, R. P. 1977. *Regional Cults.* London: Academic Press.

———. 1989. *Ritual Passage Sacred Journey: The Process and Organization of Religious Movement.* Washington, D.C.: Smithsonian Institution Press.

Wild, H. 1972. *A Rhodesian Botanical Dictionary of African and English Plant Names.* Revised and enlarged by H. M. Biegel and S. Mavi. Salisbury: Government Printers.

Wolf, C. 1980. *A Model Childhood,* translated by U. Molinaro and H. Rappolt. London: Virago. First published in German, 1976.

Wyllie, R. W. 1982. "Introspective Witchcraft among the Effutu." In *Witchcraft and Sorcery,* edited by M. Marwick. Harmondsworth, Middlesex: Penguin.

ZINATHA (Zimbabwe National Traditional Healers' Association). 1981. *Register of Traditional Medical Practitioners of Zimbabwe, 1980.* Harare: ZINATHA.

———. 1989. Survey of Traditional Healers in Zimbabwe. Unpublished document.

A NOTE ABOUT THE AUTHOR

PAMELA REYNOLDS has worked as a Social Anthropologist with children in the Zambezi Valley and Mashonaland in Zimbabwe, and in Crossroads in South Africa. She is a citizen of Zimbabwe and is currently head of the department of Social Anthropology at the University of Cape Town. Her most recent research has been with young political activists in South Africa.